COMMUNITY VIOLENCE AS A POPULATION HEALTH ISSUE

Proceedings of a Workshop

Darla Thompson and Joe Alper, *Rapporteurs*

Roundtable on Population Health Improvement

Board on Population Health and Public Health Practice

Health and Medicine Division

The National Academies of
SCIENCES · ENGINEERING · MEDICINE

THE NATIONAL ACADEMIES PRESS
Washington, DC
www.nap.edu

THE NATIONAL ACADEMIES PRESS 500 Fifth Street, NW Washington, DC 20001

This activity was supported by contracts between the National Academy of Sciences and the Aetna Foundation, The California Endowment (#10002009), Fannie E. Rippel Foundation, Health Resources and Services Administration (DHHS-10002817), New York State Health Foundation (#10001272), and Robert Wood Johnson Foundation (#10001270). Any opinions, findings, conclusions, or recommendations expressed in this publication do not necessarily reflect the views of any organization or agency that provided support for the project.

International Standard Book Number-13: 978-0-309-45047-8
International Standard Book Number-10: 0-309-45047-0
Digital Object Identifier: https://doi.org/10.17226/23661

Additional copies this publication are available for sale from the National Academies Press, 500 Fifth Street, NW, Keck 360, Washington, DC 20001; (800) 624-6242 or (202) 334-3313; http://www.nap.edu.

Printed in the United States of America

Suggested citation: National Academies of Sciences, Engineering, and Medicine. 2017. *Community violence as a population health issue: Proceedings of a workshop*. Washington, DC: The National Academies Press. doi: https://doi.org/10.17226/23661.

The National Academies of

SCIENCES · ENGINEERING · MEDICINE

The **National Academy of Sciences** was established in 1863 by an Act of Congress, signed by President Lincoln, as a private, nongovernmental institution to advise the nation on issues related to science and technology. Members are elected by their peers for outstanding contributions to research. Dr. Marcia McNutt is president.

The **National Academy of Engineering** was established in 1964 under the charter of the National Academy of Sciences to bring the practices of engineering to advising the nation. Members are elected by their peers for extraordinary contributions to engineering. Dr. C. D. Mote, Jr., is president.

The **National Academy of Medicine** (formerly the Institute of Medicine) was established in 1970 under the charter of the National Academy of Sciences to advise the nation on medical and health issues. Members are elected by their peers for distinguished contributions to medicine and health. Dr. Victor J. Dzau is president.

The three Academies work together as the **National Academies of Sciences, Engineering, and Medicine** to provide independent, objective analysis and advice to the nation and conduct other activities to solve complex problems and inform public policy decisions. The National Academies also encourage education and research, recognize outstanding contributions to knowledge, and increase public understanding in matters of science, engineering, and medicine.

Learn more about the National Academies of Sciences, Engineering, and Medicine at **www.national-academies.org**.

The National Academies of
SCIENCES • ENGINEERING • MEDICINE

Reports document the evidence-based consensus of an authoring committee of experts. Reports typically include findings, conclusions, and recommendations based on information gathered by the committee and committee deliberations. Reports are peer reviewed and are approved by the National Academies of Sciences, Engineering, and Medicine.

Proceedings chronicle the presentations and discussions at a workshop, symposium, or other convening event. The statements and opinions contained in proceedings are those of the participants and have not been endorsed by other participants, the planning committee, or the National Academies of Sciences, Engineering, and Medicine.

For information about other products and activities of the National Academies, please visit nationalacademies.org/whatwedo.

PLANNING COMMITTEE ON COMMUNITY VIOLENCE AS A POPULATION HEALTH ISSUE[1]

THOMAS LAVEIST (*Chair*), Professor and Chair, Health Policy and Management, Milken Institute School of Public Health, The George Washington University
THEODORE CORBIN, Associate Professor, Department of Emergency Medicine, Drexel University College of Medicine
RACHEL DAVIS, Managing Director, Prevention Institute
AMANDA GELLER, Clinical Associate Professor of Sociology, New York University
MARTHE R. GOLD, Visiting Scholar, The New York Academy of Medicine
GARY GUNDERSON, Vice President of Faith & Health Ministries, Medical Center Administration; Professor, Social Sciences & Health Policy, Wake Forest School of Medicine
JOHN RICH, Professor, Dornsife School of Public Health, Drexel University
THERESE S. RICHMOND, Andrea B. Laporte Professor of Nursing and Associate Dean for Research and Innovation, School of Nursing, University of Pennsylvania
LOURDES RODRÍGUEZ, Program Officer, New York State Health Foundation
DANIEL WEBSTER, Professor, Johns Hopkins Bloomberg School of Public Health; Director, Johns Hopkins Center for Gun Policy and Research; Deputy Director for Research, Johns Hopkins Center for the Prevention of Youth Violence

[1] The National Academies of Sciences, Engineering, and Medicine's planning committees are solely responsible for organizing the workshop, identifying topics, and choosing speakers. The responsibility for the published Proceedings of a Workshop rests with the workshop rapporteurs and the institution.

ROUNDTABLE ON POPULATION HEALTH IMPROVEMENT[1]

[1] The National Academies of Sciences, Engineering, and Medicine's forums and roundtables do not issue, review, or approve individual documents. The responsibility for the published Proceedings of a Workshop rests with the workshop rapporteurs and the institution.

Reviewers

This Proceedings of a Workshop was reviewed in draft form by individuals chosen for their diverse perspectives and technical expertise. The purpose of this independent review is to provide candid and critical comments that will assist the institution in making its published Proceedings of a Workshop as sound as possible and to ensure that the Proceedings of a Workshop meets institutional standards for objectivity, evidence, and responsiveness to the study charge. The review comments and draft manuscript remain confidential to protect the integrity of the process. We wish to thank the following individuals for their review of this Proceedings of a Workshop:

Delores Jones-Brown, John Jay College of Criminal Justice, City University of New York
Desmond Patton, Columbia University
Amanda Stylianou, Safe Horizon
Mark A. Zimmerman, University of Michigan, Ann Arbor

Although the reviewers listed above have provided many constructive comments and suggestions, they did not see the final draft of the Proceedings of a Workshop before its release. The review of this Proceedings of a Workshop was overseen by **Ned Calonge,** The Colorado Trust. He was responsible for making certain that an independent examination of this Proceedings of a Workshop was carried out in accordance with institutional procedures and that all review comments were carefully considered. Responsibility for the final content of this Proceedings of a Workshop rests entirely with the rapporteurs and the institution.

Acknowledgments

The sponsors of the Roundtable on Population Health Improvement have made it possible to plan and conduct "Community Violence as a Population Health Issue: A Workshop," which this Proceedings of a Workshop summarizes. Federal sponsorship was provided by the Health Resources and Services Administration. Non-federal sponsorship was provided by the Aetna Foundation, The California Endowment, New York State Health Foundation, Rippel Foundation, and the Robert Wood Johnson Foundation.

The roundtable wishes to express its appreciation to the following speakers at the workshop for their engaging and informative presentations: DeVone Boggan, Advance Peace; Charles Branas, University of Pennsylvania; Jeffrey Butts, John Jay College of Criminal Justice; Medina Howard, Center for Court Innovation; Thea James, Boston Medical Center; Steve Marans, Yale School of Medicine; John Markovic, U.S. Department of Justice; Howard Pinderhughes, University of California, San Francisco, School of Nursing; John Rich, Dornsife School of Public Health, Drexel University; Roberto Rodríguez, Stand Up to Violence at Jacobi Medical Center; and Daniel Webster, Johns Hopkins Bloomberg School of Public Health.

The roundtable also wishes to express its thanks to the planning committee for its knowledge and enthusiasm in arranging the workshop: Thomas LaVeist (*Chair*), Milken Institute School of Public Health, The George Washington University; Theodore Corbin, Department of Emergency Medicine, Drexel University College of Medicine; Rachel Davis,

Prevention Institute; Amanda Geller, New York University; Marthe R. Gold, The New York Academy of Medicine; Gary Gunderson, Wake Forest School of Medicine; John Rich, Dornsife School of Public Health, Drexel University; Therese S. Richmond, School of Nursing, University of Pennsylvania; Lourdes Rodríguez, New York State Health Foundation; and Daniel Webster, Johns Hopkins Bloomberg School of Public Health.

The roundtable also extends its thanks to Brenda Grandell, a member of the Board of Trustees at Lutheran Medical Center, and Rev. Don Stiger, the senior vice president, Mission and Spiritual Care, New York University Lutheran Medical Center. They both provided crucial assistance to the staff by making it possible to hold the workshop in a community setting at the Lutheran Church of the Good Shepherd in Brooklyn, New York.

Contents

Boxes, Figures, and Table

BOXES

FIGURES

TABLE

Acronyms and Abbreviations

ACA	Patient Protection and Affordable Care Act
ACE	adverse childhood experience
CDC	Centers for Disease Control and Prevention
COPS	Office of Community Oriented Policing Services
DOJ	U.S. Department of Justice
IOM	Institute of Medicine
NIH	National Institutes of Health
OMB	Office of Management and Budget
PTSD	posttraumatic stress disorder
RWJF	Robert Wood Johnson Foundation
SUV	Stand Up to Violence
VIAP	Violence Intervention Advocacy Program

1

Introduction[1]

On June 16, 2016, the Roundtable on Population Health Improvement held a workshop at the Lutheran Church of the Good Shepherd in Brooklyn, New York, to explore the influence of trauma and violence on communities.[2] George Isham, co-chair of the roundtable, welcomed participants and explained that hanging behind the podium was a peace quilt created by children of the church congregation. The quilt included several quotes, such as "Love and Open Your Hearts to Others" and "Peace Begins with Me." Isham pointed out that this was a significant backdrop, both physically and metaphorically for the conversation of the day. As participants were painfully aware, though the workshop on community violence as a population health issue had been in the planning stages for several weeks, just a few days earlier, on June 12, 2016, Omar Mateen shot and killed 49 people and injured 53 others at Pulse, a gay nightclub located in Orlando, Florida. Isham said

---

[1] The planning committee's role was limited to planning the workshop, and the Proceedings of a Workshop was prepared by the workshop rapporteurs as a factual summary of what occurred at the workshop. Statements, recommendations, and opinions expressed are those of individual presenters and participants, and have not been endorsed or verified by the National Academies of Sciences, Engineering, and Medicine, and they should not be construed as reflecting any group consensus.

[2] The workshop was held at the Lutheran Church of the Good Shepherd because the planning committee was interested in holding this workshop in a non-academic setting. Gary Gunderson, a member of the roundtable and planning committee, introduced staff to Dan Stiger of the New York University Lutheran Medical Center who recommended the Lutheran Church of the Good Shepherd.

it was appropriate to keep this tragic national event and the loss of lives and injured people in mind, as well as to think of the families, loved ones, and others in the community affected by this violence.

In his introductory comments, Isham said that since February 2013, the roundtable has served as a venue for leaders to meet and discuss the leverage points and opportunities arising from changes in the social and political environment for advancing better population health. At previous workshops held by the roundtable, "The Role and Potential of Communities in Population Health Improvement: A Workshop" (IOM, 2015) and "Supporting a Movement for Health and Health Equity: Lessons from Social Movements: A Workshop" (IOM, 2014), several individual workshop speakers emphasized that safe and healthy communities are central to health equity and improving population health. Individual speakers also conveyed the message that community engagement and organizing are important approaches to addressing the social determinants of health, such as housing, education, and violence. Isham added that also relevant was the workshop "Framing the Dialogue on Race and Ethnicity to Advance Health Equity: A Workshop" (NASEM, 2016b), in which Gilbert C. Gee discussed how racism contributes to shorter lives for people of color and inequities in life expectancy. This workshop builds on those insights and seeks to explore ways in which communities are addressing violence and building safe, healthy, and resilient communities.

WORKSHOP OBJECTIVES

An important activity of the roundtable is to hold workshops for its members, stakeholders, and the public to discuss issues that contribute to improving the nation's health. An independent planning committee, chaired by Thomas LaVeist, and including Theodore Corbin, Rachel Davis, Amanda Geller, Marthe Gold, Gary Gunderson, John Rich, Therese Richmond, Lourdes Rodríguez, and Daniel Webster, was charged with developing a workshop to explore community violence and trauma through a health equity lens (see Box 1-1). The workshop was designed to

- explore the impacts of trauma and violence on communities;
- explore strategies and approaches that communities and multisector partners are using to reduce violence and build resilience;
- explore the evidence base for the effectiveness of strategies and approaches for reducing the impact of violence on communities; and
- provide a platform for programs and initiatives that can serve as models for other communities, with an explicit attention to the intersections of structural racism and structural violence.

BOX 1-1
Statement of Task

An ad hoc committee will plan and convene a public workshop exploring trauma-informed approaches to community violence through a health equity lens. The committee will develop the agenda and identify meeting objectives, select appropriate speakers, and moderate the discussions. The workshop may highlight and explore examples of community-based organizations using trauma-informed approaches to treat violence and build safe and healthy communities; strategies to build resilience in children, adults, and communities; hospital and health system violence intervention programs; trauma-informed policing; and the evidence base for the effectiveness of these strategies and approaches to reducing violence and its impact on communities. The workshop intends to showcase examples that can serve as models in different sectors and communities and share lessons learned in new and compelling ways. A summary of the presentations and discussions at the workshop will be prepared by a designated rapporteur in accordance with institutional guidelines.

As explained by LaVeist of The George Washington University, while the tragic shooting at the Pulse nightclub in Orlando makes this seem like a particularly fitting topic to address, it is also the case that given the amount of violence that occurs every day in this country, it is appropriate any day to discuss this topic. The planning committee presented a broad range of concerns to the roundtable, such as police violence, gun violence, and trauma-informed community building, and recent work of the National Academies of Sciences, Engineering, and Medicine (e.g., IOM and NRC, 2013a,b; IOM, 2015; and NASEM, 2015).[3] Members thought it was most appropriate to focus the workshop on community violence and innovative approaches to building resilient communities. Therefore, the planning committee decided this workshop should be attentive to the everyday structural violence that disproportionately affects communities of color living in poverty.

"We know that violence is a social determinant of health," said LaVeist. Violence is a factor—along with racism; toxic stress; lack of access to healthy food; poor quality or no housing; lack of adequate education,

[3] Many publications by the National Academies' Forum on Global Violence Prevention are available at http://www.nationalacademies.org/hmd/Reports.aspx?filters=inmeta:activity=Forum+on+Global+Violence+Prevention (accessed October 31, 2016). Publications from the Committee on Law and Justice and other units are also available at http://sites.nationalacademies.org/DBASSE/CLAJ/Topics/DBASSE_080822 (accessed October 31, 2016).

jobs, and incomes; and lack of safe places to walk, play, and socialize—that shapes the health of individuals and communities and contributes to shorter lives, particularly for people of color, he added. The planning committee intended for this workshop to be a way to bring attention within the population health field to the problem of public acts of violence and its corrosive effects on health, safety, and the well-being of individuals and communities across the nation. This Proceedings of a Workshop is not intended as a comprehensive summary of the science and evidence on community violence as a population health issue. The initiatives, organizations, academic institutions, and individuals featured in this workshop are only a few of the many considered by the planning committee. Participants' inclusion in the workshop was based on a range of factors, none of which is related to privileging or promoting particular approaches or programs over others.[4]

Two topics were mentioned by several workshop participants during the discussions throughout the day for their absence: (1) a focus on violence against lesbian, gay, bisexual, transgender, queer, and questioning (LGBTQ) communities; and (2) a focus on domestic violence against women and children. Planning committee members did discuss community violence as public acts of violence,[5] and members of the planning committee who participated at the workshop acknowledged and welcomed the comments about the lack of focus on the relationship between intimate partner violence by men against women involved in gun violence (see discussion sections in Chapters 4, 5, and 7). Also welcome were the comments about the lack of focus on violence against LGBTQ communities, particularly during the reflections at the end of the day (see Chapter 7).

ORGANIZATION OF THE PROCEEDINGS

This Proceedings of a Workshop synthesizes the discussions that occurred during the workshop, highlights the speakers' perspectives on community violence as a population health issue, and discusses some of

---

[4] The draft resource list developed by staff as background reading for the workshop includes information on many additional violence prevention initiatives, though it was also not intended to be comprehensive, but rather illustrative of national initiatives. It is available at the activity page for the workshop at the website of the Roundtable on Population Health Improvement, see http://nationalacademies.org/hmd/~/media/Files/Activity%20Files/PublicHealth/PopulationHealthImprovementRT/16-JUN-16/21%20Resource%20list.pdf (accessed October 31, 2016).

[5] Examples of definitions of community violence can be found at the following sites: http://www.nctsn.org/trauma-types/community-violence (accessed September 16, 2016) and http://www.cvtcnyc.org/communityviolence (accessed September 16, 2016).

the strategies communities are using to reduce violence and the impact of violence. Chapter 2 discusses the impact of racism and violence on communities. Chapter 3 describes some social and physical interventions that can change landscapes of violence, and Chapter 4 addresses local strategies to build community resilience and safety. Chapter 5 discusses some lessons learned from select approaches and initiatives designed to reduce community violence, and Chapter 6 explores public health–informed approaches to community policing and collaboration. Chapter 7 provides a reflection on the day's presentations and discussions.

In accordance with the policies of the National Academies of Sciences, Engineering, and Medicine, workshop participants did not attempt to establish any conclusions or recommendations about needs and future directions, focusing instead on issues identified by the speakers and workshop participants. In addition, the planning committee's role was limited to planning the workshop. The Proceedings of a Workshop was prepared by workshop rapporteurs Darla Thompson and Joe Alper as a factual summary of what occurred at the workshop.

2

The Impact of Racism and Violence on Communities[1]

The workshop opened with a keynote presentation by John A. Rich, professor at the Dornsife School of Public Health, Drexel University. He noted that although mass shootings such as the one on June 12, 2016, in Orlando, Florida, get the nation's attention, acts of violence—homicides, shootings, aggravated assaults, and others—are everyday events in too many communities across the country. Asked by the planning committee to begin a conversation about racism and violence and their impacts on communities, Rich said the goal of his presentation was to create a sense of hope. "When you are talking about violence and racism, it can sometimes seem overwhelming in terms of what we need to do," said Rich, "but I hope, at the end, that we get to the point where we recognize that by addressing violence in the context of inequality, we move toward something more than simply reducing violence. We move toward greater health equity." Highlights of Rich's presentation are in Box 2-1.

To illustrate the problem, Rich cited data on the number of homicides, shootings, and aggravated assaults in Philadelphia and New York (see Figure 2-1). These figures show that while violence is often tracked in terms of homicides, murder represents just a small fraction of the violence in affected communities. Moreover, those figures do not account for assaults that are not reported to the police, nor do they measure the

[1] This chapter is the rapporteurs' synopsis of the presentation made by John A. Rich, professor at the Drexel University Dornsife School of Public Health, and the statements have not been endorsed or verified by the National Academies of Sciences, Engineering, and Medicine.

BOX 2-1
Highlights of Keynote Presentation Made by John Rich[a]

- Regardless of the framework, violence is a public health issue.
- There are tremendous disparities in the ways in which violence affects communities.
- Police violence against young people of color has become a critical factor in how the nation thinks about the violence happening in communities.
- One might argue that young people of color need the police as much or more than any other group, so intrusive violence encounters designed to keep the community safe often have a negative consequence instead.
- A trauma-informed framework might suggest ways of interrupting the cycle of young men of color believing that using firearms is the way to protect themselves from violence.
- The health system can intervene in a way that is consistent with a trauma-informed framework, said Rich. However, it cannot avoid dealing with racism given the health care system's past display of historic institutional racism, and the fact that there are disparities in medical care and a lack of diversity among health care providers.
- All the efforts to reduce violence are not enough if there is not also an effort to address health equity.

[a] This list is the rapporteurs' summary of the main points made by the keynote speaker, and the statements have not been endorsed or verified by the National Academies of Sciences, Engineering, and Medicine.

impact on a child who has to walk past yellow crime scene tape on the way to school or on the grandmother sitting on her porch who wonders if the gunfire she just heard had something to do with a family member. "The scope of violence and trauma goes far beyond these numbers and the specific medical or public health issues that we see, and that means trauma is really at the heart of what we are thinking about in terms of violence," said Rich.

There are a number of frameworks from which to think about violence, said Rich. For example, violence can be viewed through the lens of trauma, but it can also be seen in terms of contagion, learned behavior, or addiction. Some people consider violence a mental illness or a moral defect, or in terms of a culture of violence. Regardless of the framework, however, violence is a public health issue, said Rich, and he suggested these frameworks are not mutually exclusive. As an example, he said that violence might be seen as contagious with the agent being trauma. Not all combinations are useful, though—the view of violence as a combination of learned behavior and moral defect, he added, led to the development of ineffective programs such as Scared Straight.

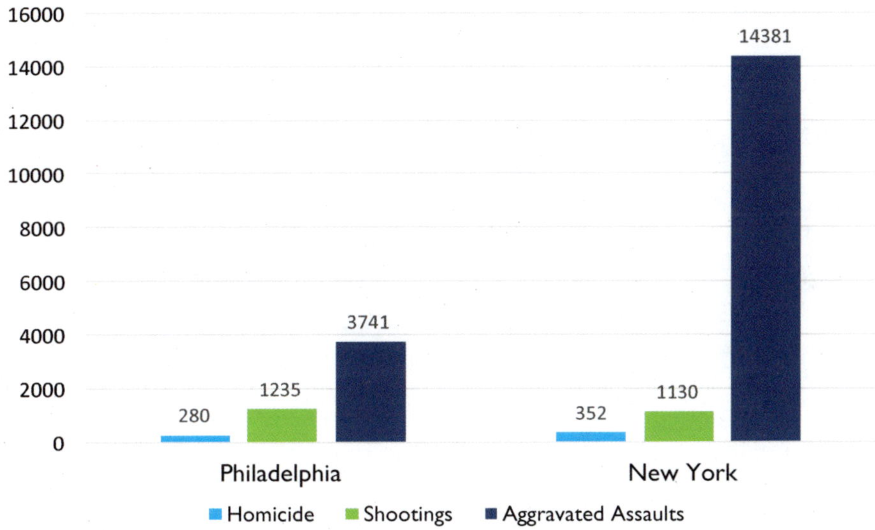

FIGURE 2-1 Violence in Philadelphia and New York City, 2015.
SOURCE: Rich presentation, June 16, 2016.

Many commentators use the "war zone" metaphor to portray communities affected by violence, but Rich said the loss these communities feel may be larger than in actual war zones. Between 2001 and 2010, for example, 1,446 American soldiers lost their lives fighting in Afghanistan and 4,400 were killed serving in Iraq. Over that same period, 3,391 people were murdered in Philadelphia. "So in one U.S. city, the order of magnitude of loss is tremendous," said Rich, who added that there are tremendous disparities in the ways in which violence affects communities. He noted, too, that over the same 10-year period, 45,416 African American males under the age of 34 were killed by gunfire in the United States.

Race, however, should not be the focus of the discussion about violence, said Rich. "We know that race is a social construction. We know that race does not bear any reality in terms of biology, that it is just a phenotypic manifestation," said Rich. "Therefore, whenever we see this kind of disparity, it is not enough to talk about, for example, Black-on-Black violence as though that is an answer to a question." Instead, he said, it is important to understand that race is serving as a proxy for the real cause, be that poverty, disadvantage, or disparity. He cited a study (Feldmeyer, 2010) in which the author concluded that racial and ethnic segregation contributes to the elevated rates of homicide among both Latinos and

African Americans and that the effects for both groups are mediated by concentrated disadvantage.

In addition to the number of frameworks for thinking about violence, there are various frameworks for looking at racism. The framework developed by Camara Jones (Jones, 2002) defines racism as a system of structuring opportunity and assigning value based on phenotype that unfairly disadvantages some individuals and communities, unfairly advantages other individuals and communities, and saps the strength of the whole society through the waste of human resources. According to this framework, racism has more than one effect in that it does not merely disadvantage those affected by it, but gives advantage to others, which in the context of violence means there are some young people who are more likely to be victimized and others who are less likely to be victimized because of privilege and birth position, said Rich. "We must account both for what is lost and what is gained in thinking about racism," he said.

This framework for racism also includes three levels at which racism functions (Jones, 2000). The first is institutional racism, defined as the differential access to the goods, services, and opportunities of society by race. Institutional racism, said Rich, explains the association between social class and race. The next level, personally mediated racism, is what is often thought of when discussing racism, and it is defined as the differential assumptions about the abilities, motives, and intents of others by race—prejudice—or the differential actions based on those assumptions, that is, discrimination. This framework holds that institutional racism is mediated through individuals. The third level of racism is internalized racism, which represents that acceptance by the stigmatized races of negative messages about their own abilities and intrinsic worth.

Turning to the recent attention focused on police violence and racism, Rich said police violence against young people of color has become a critical factor in how the nation thinks about the violence happening in communities. Police violence against people of color is not new, but Rich believes it has only now grabbed the public's attention because it is being captured on mobile phones and played back for all to see. As examples, he recounted Rodney King's brutal beating in 1991, Abner Louima's brutalization and torture by New York City police in 1997, the 1999 shooting of Amadou Diallo when police mistook his wallet for a gun as he was entering his home, and Sean Bell, the young groom who was shot 50 times by police on the day of his wedding in 2006. Rich said it is likely that between 2006 and 2012, when Trayvon Martin was killed by a vigilante in his Sanford, Florida, neighborhood, that there were other black male children and adults killed in the United States in a similar manner not brought to the public's attention. Since then, however, the police-involved deaths of Michael Brown, Eric Garner, Freddie Gray, Laquan McDonald,

Tamir Rice, and Walter Scott have reinforced the notion that young people may not see the police as a protective force.

Applying the racism framework, Rich said police violence requires first thinking about the relationship between historical discrimination and institutional racism. He noted that in 2015, the police commissioner of New York City said, "Slavery, our country's original sin, sat on a foundation codified by laws enforced by police, by slave catchers." Today, said Rich, institutional racism is seen in the police policies that legitimize and even incentivize aggressive action against young men of color, with "stop and frisk" policies and racial profiling as examples. Rich recounted an incident in Philadelphia that involved the police being called by a ticket agent who said a young man did not pay his fare to board a train. In a surveillance video, an African American transit police officer has his hands around the neck of the young African American man who was holding a child. This incident is illustrative of institutional racism, said Rich, because in explaining what happened, the head of the transit police said the officer believed it was his duty to act that way or he would be disciplined for violating policy. This may also be an example of the internalized racism of the African American police officer, Rich said.

What is also powerful about this example, said Rich, is that a young child was impacted by police violence. "In this day where we talk more and more about early childhood adversity and its impact later in people's lives, we know that police officers often encounter families in settings where there are children and where what they are doing will serve as a traumatizing effect on that child that may have a future impact on that child's health and the family's health," said Rich.

Personally mediated racism can then lead to the dehumanizing treatment of young men of color driven by implicit bias, instances of which Rich said he heard in the interviews he and his colleagues have done with hundreds of young people who have been victims of violence in their communities. One young man from Boston, for example, was shot when a robber tried to take his chain and he recalled the police officer saying, "Don't do nothin' stupid like die." Often, young people said they were verbally assaulted in an attempt to get information from them when they were injured. Rich said these young people understand that police have a role to play in apprehending the individuals responsible for the violence, but these types of encounters stick in their minds.

Internalized racism is apparent in the aggressive and violent acts by police officers of color toward young people, and these acts, said Rich, can have an impact that goes beyond what happens in the streets. One study found, for example, that participants who reported more police contact, particularly intrusive police contact, experienced more symptoms of trauma and anxiety (Geller et al., 2014). The associations were tied to how many stops the individuals reported, the intrusiveness of the encounters, and their perceptions of police fairness. Another study found that young people who have had contact with the criminal justice system are more likely to avoid interacting with that system in the future (Brayne, 2014). This latter finding is important, said Rich, because young men of color have the highest victimization rates of any group. "One might argue they need the police as much or more than any other group, so these encounters designed to keep the community safe often have a negative consequence," he explained.

After showing a video of Dave Green,[2] a client of Healing Hurt People[3] recounting the impact that his multiple experiences with violence have had on his health and well-being, Rich said some might listen to that story and say the young man was living in a culture of violence. However, looking at this young man's experiences through a trauma-informed lens would suggest he is experiencing the classic symptoms of posttraumatic stress disorder (PTSD) and depression that sends him into a spiral of feeling unsafe. Rich noted one study's findings that nearly three-quarters of the victims of violence have high rates of PTSD (Corbin et al., 2013), but another study at the Boston Medical Center found that 23 percent of the patients in a primary care clinic had PTSD, though that diagnosis was recorded in only 11 percent of the cases (Liebschutz et al., 2007).

Research has also shown violence to be a chronic, recurrent disease. Studies in Chicago and Baltimore found that 44 percent of the individuals who had experienced a penetrating injury were injured again over the next 5 years and 20 percent of those individuals were dead. These data, Rich said, show that "efforts that focus on health care environments or places where victims are seen have to be part of a broader solution for interrupting the cycle of violence."

A common image among those who work in medical settings is that someone repeatedly injured is involved in activities that predispose that person to violence, said Rich. However, when Rich and his colleagues talked to young people, they found that this is not a reliable way to think about their lives. Instead, a trauma-informed approach takes the view that a young person who has been injured and has PTSD or other symptoms of trauma is rarely informed they may experience those symptoms. As a result, when that youth has nightmares and flashbacks, and feels as if he or she is going crazy and turns to whatever is available in the environ-

[2] Dave Green's digital story may be viewed as part of John Rich's presentation at http://www.nationalacademies.org/hmd/Activities/PublicHealth/PopulationHealthImprovementRT/2016-JUN-16/Videos/Welcome/2-Rich-Video.aspx (accessed September 12, 2016).

[3] For more information, see http://www.nonviolenceandsocialjustice.org/Healing-Hurt-People/29 (accessed August 18, 2016).

ment to treat his or her distress, in communities lacking access to health care, what is available is often alcohol or marijuana.

For a young person of color living in the inner city, said Rich, access to marijuana in particular often means that individual will have limited access to employment, particularly for entry-level jobs that require drug testing. It also means they are more likely to have contact with law enforcement and the criminal justice system, which places them in the world of mass incarceration that leads to other negative downstream effects, said Rich.

One consequence of young men of color's general distrust of law enforcement, Rich explained, is that they are more likely to own a firearm in order to protect themselves. Having a weapon, however, then increases the odds of experiencing further trauma and even death. "A trauma-informed framework might suggest ways of interrupting this cycle," said Rich.

Rich and his colleagues developed Healing Hurt People, a hospital-based, trauma-informed, community-focused violence intervention program for victims of violence who are at high risk of further exposure to violence. After their discharge from the hospital, victims of violence are assigned to social work staff and outreach workers who assess the person's living arrangements and environment to determine if they are at risk or safe. An individual having symptoms of trauma is invited to enroll in a trauma-informed program that includes a deeper assessment, case management, and navigation to systems that may be otherwise inaccessible to these young people. Youth also receive mentoring, powerful group interventions in which young people have the opportunity to process their trauma, and where needed, more specific therapy.

The health system can intervene in a way that is consistent with a trauma-informed framework, said Rich. However, it cannot avoid dealing with racism given the health care system's past display of historic institutional racism, such as the Tuskegee Experiment[4] and Jim Crow segregation in hospitals, and the fact that there are disparities in medical care and a lack of diversity among health care providers. Individuals of color also report examples of personally mediated racism such as disrespectful treatment by health care providers and the phenomenon of mistaken identity, in which health care providers are mistaken for custodial staff, experiences that some may call microaggressions. There may also be internalized racism that manifests in persons of color preferring white providers because they have come to believe that providers of color could not possibly be as good as their white counterparts.

---

[4] For more information, see http://www.cdc.gov/tuskegee/timeline.htm (accessed September 12, 2016).

Given that this is the context in which violence occurs, Rich explained how they can incorporate these insights into trauma-informed approaches to violence and racism. The first step is to acknowledge the historical racism in medicine and health care. To deal with institutional racism, he and his colleagues convene quarterly gatherings of the leaders of health systems in Philadelphia that serve these young people, and present a case to them so they can begin to think about structural barriers. They also collect data and engage community health workers who are more likely to be aware of institutional racism.

Rich and his team address personally mediated racism through implicit bias training for staff and residents that includes having clients reflect on their experiences of racism. To address internalized racism, one approach that Rich's team uses is engaging young victims in trauma-informed dialog about racism as a trauma in addition to training them to be community health workers. After receiving their training, the youth then share their experiences with other members of the health care team.[5]

In conclusion, Rich said, "In all of our efforts, we should be seeking to reduce violence, but it is not enough to reduce violence if we are not also addressing health equity." Addressing health equity requires a different level of resources, he added, because these young people are for the most part not plugged into what he called the grid of opportunity. "Young people of color often need help plugging into that grid of opportunity so that they can thrive and so that their health can improve and we can begin to address the social determinants of health," said Rich. The outcomes and benefits of devoting those extra resources, he added, will accrue to public health beyond reducing violence in affected communities.

As a final note, he stated that firearms remain a tremendous challenge. The Institute of Medicine and the National Research Council have articulated a set of priorities for firearms research (IOM and NRC, 2013b), and Rich called on those at the workshop to put forth as forcefully as possible the idea that firearm-mediated violence is a health equity issue.

DISCUSSION

Thomas LaVeist of The George Washington University opened the discussion by asking Rich to address the issue of violence as an adaptive behavior. Rich acknowledged the importance of that view and said the research community has begun to think more about some of these behaviors as reactions that are logical in the sense that if these young people see the horizon of possibilities as limited, if they do not see the police as protecting them, if they are hyperaroused by trauma, and if they live in

[5] For more information on Healing Hurt People, see http://www.nonviolenceandsocialjustice.org/Healing-Hurt-People/29 (accessed November 1, 2016).

communities that speak to them about the danger they face, then getting a weapon is a logical, potentially adaptive way to stay safe. One thing Rich has heard from the young people he has interviewed who live in a hostile environment is that if they allow someone to victimize them and do not respond, they are sending a message to the community that they are going to continue to be victims. This is certainly not a new idea invented by these young people, said Rich, but when it plays out in places where there is a sense of limited opportunities, young people are forced to stand their ground. "If caring adults do not step up when you are getting beat up for your lunch money, you learn after a few times you better stand up for yourself," said Rich.

LaVeist then asked Rich to describe an intervention based on a framework that people are acting violently as a violence prevention strategy. Rich replied that such an intervention needs to start by helping young people understand the impact of trauma in shaping whether they can judge what is safe and not safe. "Anyone who is traumatized and hyperaroused may not be able to distinguish life-threatening threats from non-life-threatening threats, and I think that is why we often hear about flashpoints," said Rich, referring to seemingly innocuous events leading to violence. Another piece of an intervention would be to help young people think about what would be reasonable alternatives in their communities, and when there are not reasonable alternatives, engage them in a process of fashioning solutions. "One thing we know is that people who survive trauma often come away with what we call a survivor mission," said Rich. "They are motivated to do something to induce change." Tapping into that motivation and connecting with the potential consequences for the community can have a real impact, Rich explained, but only if there are opportunities for work and if the affected individuals can see those opportunities. Too often, institutional racism cuts young people off from those opportunities if they have had an encounter with the criminal justice system.

Sanne Magnan asked Rich about the bind African American police officers may feel when dealing with an African American youth. This bind, said Rich, is related to what he called stereotype threat, where individuals feel they are representing not just themselves, but others as well. In the case of an African American police officer, he or she may feel that it will reflect poorly if they somehow give a break to the young person they are confronting. Addressing this problem, said Rich, takes a full and comprehensive institutional assessment to find all of the policies and practices that perpetuate institutional racism and then instituting new training and hiring practices. The problem is that the solutions proposed to these kinds of dilemmas are often focused on the individual officer rather than at the system level, Rich added.

George Isham of HealthPartners wondered if Rich had ideas for remedies that can begin dealing with the cascade of factors involved in racism, from institutional to internalized, that reinforce each other. Commenting that Isham is right that these are all interconnected, Rich said any intervention needs to work at all levels, must include input from the community, and must be broad-based and comprehensive.

Raymond Baxter of Kaiser Permanente commented that the United States has been at war in one country or another for decades and asked Rich, given the violence as war framework he mentioned, if there are consequences with regard to violence in America. Rich responded that this was a profound question, and explained that when he used the metaphor of violence as war, he was thinking about communities feeling besieged in the way people living in war zones feel. The way war is depicted reinforces the notion that there is a differential value of human life, and within the United States, many people come to accept that young people of color are dying every day, in contrast to the way the nation reacts to a major event or a natural disaster that kills hundreds or thousands of people. There is a need to understand that human life is valuable regardless of how opportunity is "sliced and diced" in this society, said Rich.

Daniel Webster of the Johns Hopkins Bloomberg School of Public Health commented that the War on Drugs has had an outsized impact on disadvantaged communities of color and in his opinion, reforming drug laws should be a central part of any population health approach to reducing violence in those communities. Rich said that was "absolutely right," though he noted that the police have had a negative impact on communities of color long before the War on Drugs. Still, he said, it is obvious that the nation's drug policies have been applied disproportionately in terms of penalties and enforcement. Undoing those policies is a start, but the racism underlying those policies needs to be addressed, too, said Rich.

Catherine Baase of The Dow Chemical Company asked Rich to comment on the nation's capacity to advance a framework of peace at a societal level. Rich replied that he and his colleagues think a great deal about nonviolence and how to engage young people in conversations about what nonviolence means. He noted that engaging the nation in a framework of peace requires accepting the fact that the United States is a great consumer of violence. "Violence sells. We are engaged in it. The rest of the world looks at us and cannot quite understand, so we have to reckon with this," said Rich. He noted that there are models across the world for creating equitable and more peaceful societies, and the question is whether or not the United States is willing to engage in those models. Doing so, he added, requires moving beyond an "us and them" perspective on violence even though it disproportionately affects particular populations.

3

Changing Landscapes of Violence Through Social and Physical Interventions

The workshop's first panel session began with moderator Therese S. Richmond, the Andrea B. Laporte Professor of Nursing and associate dean for research and innovation at the University of Pennsylvania School of Nursing, describing four take-home points from the research she and her team have conducted on the strategies young people and adults use to stay safe in their communities. Howard Pinderhughes, associate professor and chair of social and behavioral sciences at the University of California, San Francisco, School of Nursing, then presented a framework he has developed with colleagues at the Prevention Institute on community trauma and resilience, and Charles Branas, professor of epidemiology and director of the Penn Injury Science Center and the Urban Health Lab at the University of Pennsylvania, discussed an evidence-based solution to firearm violence. Richmond moderated an open discussion following the presentations. Highlights and main points made by individual speakers are in Box 3-1.

STAYING SAFE IN THE COMMUNITY[1]

To set the context for the two subsequent presentations, Therese Richmond presented four briefs she prepared from the research she and

[1] This section is the rapporteurs' synopsis of the presentation made by Therese S. Richmond, the Andrea B. Laporte Professor of Nursing and associate dean for research and innovation at the University of Pennsylvania School of Nursing. The statements have

BOX 3-1
Highlights and Main Points Made by Individual Speakers[a]

- It is possible to change lives one block at a time (Richmond).
- Community trauma is not merely the aggregate of individuals in a neighborhood who have experienced trauma from exposure to violence. Rather, there are symptoms of community trauma that come from cumulative and synergistic impacts of regular experiences of interpersonal violence, of historical and intergenerational violence, and of continual exposure to structural violence (Pinderhughes).
- Dislocation and gentrification are more recent additional elements of structural violence (Pinderhughes).
- Social networks and infrastructures of social support, including culturally relevant mental health approaches, can strengthen and elevate social norms, promote healthy behaviors, and establish collaborations that promote healthy communities (Pinderhughes).
- If you can positively affect a place, the thing people see every day on their way to work, school, or play, you might do it in a way that helps people and makes things better without asking them to do anything (Branas).
- Once you change an environment by improving it, people become invested, and that changes a lot of the informal policing structures in the community (Branas).

[a] This list is the rapporteurs' summary of the main points made by individual speakers (noted in parentheses), and the statements have not been endorsed or verified by the National Academies of Sciences, Engineering, and Medicine.

her colleagues have conducted on community violence. The first came from a study in West Philadelphia examining the impact of exposure to community violence on 10- to 16-year-old children (McDonald et al., 2011). Some 95 percent of the study participants had heard about violence in their community, 87 percent had directly witnessed violent events, and 54 percent had been victimized directly. Of the latter group, one-third had been victimized two or more times. "The impact of community violence on this group of youth, from impoverished and violent communities and communities of color, was substantial," said Richmond.

The second snapshot illustrated the constant vigilance young people in violent communities maintain to cope with the stress of living in such communities (Teitelman et al., 2010). These youths, said Richmond,

not been endorsed or verified by the National Academies of Sciences, Engineering, and Medicine.

display a finely tuned and highly nuanced understanding of the risks they face in navigating their environments. While on the one hand such vigilance is not only warranted but a desirable behavior, this constant vigilance carriers a burden from an allostatic load associated with chronic stress, which Richmond explained is known to contribute significantly to increased morbidity and mortality. Indeed, she said, life expectancy for African American men and women in these communities is less than 70 years of age.

The third snapshot comes from work with long-time community partners to find out how children and parents in violent neighborhoods navigate their environments (Jacoby et al., 2016). She and her colleagues interviewed dyads of parents and children who had previously been homeless or had unstable housing and were now living in ACHIEVEability, a subsidized housing plus nonprofit in Philadelphia. This mapping exercise revealed that parents rarely permitted these 10- to 17-year-old children to leave their own homes, particularly in the summer when school was out of session, a finding Richmond called highly disturbing. Parents prioritized the safety of their children over the potential physical and mental ramifications of social isolation and inactivity (Jacoby et al., 2016). "They were not navigating their environments, so think about the health consequences of living in environments where violence is pervasive," said Richmond.

The final snapshot Richmond shared, one she said was highly relevant to why it is important to change landscapes from a social and physical perspective, looked at the effect of microneighborhood conditions on adult educational attainment because education is considered a path out of poverty. This study, again conducted with colleagues at ACHIEVEability, looked at how adults living in 130 housing units spread across a 2.1-mile radius in West Philadelphia progressed toward finishing their general educational development degree, their associate degree, and finally a bachelor's degree, all requirements for living in ACHIEVEability. These adults and their children were assigned to whatever housing unit was available at the time they entered the program (thus, quasi-random assignment), and those who lived on low-crime blocks accrued higher education credits more rapidly compared to those who lived on moderate- and high-crime blocks (Tach et al., 2016). What these results show, said Richmond, is that it is possible to change lives one block at a time.

A FRAMEWORK FOR COMMUNITY TRAUMA[2]

"I think everyone can agree that we have a number of traumatized communities across the country, particularly in our inner cities, but even in our rural neighborhoods," said Howard Pinderhughes as an introduction to his presentation about community-level approaches to healing traumatized communities. His first experience with violence in his childhood neighborhood in Roxbury, Massachusetts, occurred at age 8, when his 6-year-old neighbor's body was found in a green plastic bag sitting under the mailbox across the street from Pinderhughes's house. He was reminded of his childhood exposure to violence by a more recent incident, a gang-related shooting in 2011 that claimed an infant in West Oakland, California. Working in the community at the time, Pinderhughes observed that people who did not even know this child were impacted tremendously and were in despair. "It hit home to me that community trauma goes beyond the individual person who is traumatized, beyond even the people in the family who are impacted, so we have to think about it in much wider terms," said Pinderhughes.

Dealing with violence is not a new phenomenon for communities, said Pinderhughes. As a result, young people have been going to too many funerals and dealing for too long with the daily reality of the possibility and potential to be victims of violence. "What I have seen with the young people that I have been working with is that it has become so normalized we have a whole cottage industry that has grown up around dealing with loss," said Pinderhughes. Within hours of a violence claiming a life, T-shirts come out and shrines go up, he noted, and communities begin trying to process their loss.

Today, he said, there is a growing understanding of the impact of what are called adverse childhood experiences (ACEs).[3] The importance of ACEs was first elucidated by a joint Kaiser Permanente–Centers for Disease Control and Prevention (CDC) study of more than 17,000 Kaiser members in Southern California (Felitti et al., 1998). Conducted between 1995 and 1997, this study found that adults, largely white and middle class, who had four or more adverse childhood experiences from a list of nine were more likely to have chronic disease and suffer from a mental illness. With the young people he works with, the question Pinderhughes asks is what happens when children experience all nine of these adverse

---

[2] This section is the rapporteurs' synopsis of the presentation made by Howard Pinderhughes, associate professor and chair of social and behavioral sciences at the University of California, San Francisco, School of Nursing. The statements have not been endorsed or verified by the National Academies of Sciences, Engineering, and Medicine.

[3] For more information, see https://www.cdc.gov/violenceprevention/acestudy (accessed September 15, 2016).

experiences on a daily basis, and this led him to develop the concept of synergistic trauma.

Synergistic trauma, he explained, is the combination of individual trauma from exposures to violence and the trauma from structural violence. Structural violence refers to the harm individuals, families, and communities experience from the economic and social structure, social institutions, and relations of power, privilege, and inequity that may harm people and communities by preventing them from getting their basic needs met. The concept of synergistic trauma also integrates the concept of complex posttraumatic stress disorder, which he said is a psychological injury resulting from protracted exposure to prolonged social and interpersonal trauma in the context of either captivity or entrapment.

Although people can experience police departments as a social institution that can potentially inflect harm, they are not the only community institution in the most impacted communities that induce trauma rather than serving as foundations and developers of resilience, said Pinderhughes. Other institutions, he added, such as schools, the foster care system, and the juvenile and criminal justice systems, may also perpetuate harm. "We have all of these systems that we move our young people through as they are traumatized and what do we do? We place them in contexts that further traumatize them," said Pinderhughes. An economy and employment structure that often excludes members of the community represents another contributor to structural violence.

Pinderhughes said that the United States mass produces violence, and various root causes, environmental factors, and individual-level factors contribute to the production of violence. Most of the nation's analysis, policies, and attention, he said, are focused on the individual level, and such attention is warranted. "Part of what we have come to understand over the past 15 years is the profound impact trauma has at the individual level in terms of people's psychosocial state, their emotional state, and the motivations that they used for the behavior, particularly violent behaviors that they engage in," said Pinderhughes. Trauma, he explained, alters, shapes, and impacts the ways in which these factors affect the individual, as does structural violence and community trauma. Community trauma, said Pinderhughes, is not merely the aggregate of individuals in a neighborhood who have experienced trauma from exposure to violence. Rather, there are symptoms of community trauma that come from cumulative and synergistic impacts of regular experiences of interpersonal violence, of historical and intergenerational violence, and of the continual exposure to structural violence.

The framework Pinderhughes developed in collaboration with the Prevention Institute was constructed using the Prevention Institute's

Thrive tool,[4] which looks at three domains of a healthy community: equitable economic and educational opportunity, the physical built environment, and the social and cultural environment (Pinderhughes et al., 2015). The symptoms of community trauma occur when the community no longer functions as the fabric and foundation of resilience for young people and families exposed to both interpersonal and structural violence. Instead, the community becomes a place that helps to produce violence rather than protecting its residents from the impacts of violence. Housing projects, which become deteriorated, unhealthy places with dangerous public spaces and crumbling built environments approximating prisons, are an example of a community with none of the domains of a healthy community. Intergenerational poverty, long-term unemployment, fleeing businesses, limited local employment opportunities, and government and private disinvestment also contribute to community trauma.

Dislocation and gentrification are more recent additional elements of structural violence. "The minute we are successful in helping to transform communities, folks are dislodged and moved out," said Pinderhughes. As a result, people from these recovering communities relocate to new areas where they have the same set of problems, but with fewer services. In addition, gentrification and dislocation damage the social and cultural environments in which these individuals and families live, destroying their social networks and social support infrastructure. What follows, he said, is a low sense of collective political and social efficacy, and the elevation of destructive norms that promote violence and unhealthy behaviors instead of affirming community-oriented positive social norms. Examples include the thug and pimp cultures that develop among high schoolers in violent communities. Pinderhughes asked several questions, such as Where do the behavioral norms come from? How do we reverse them? "What happens when young people grow up in neighborhoods that are constructed as killing zones and they understand that that is their environment and that is their future?"

While research has shown that adversity can be a positive in someone's life because it helps develop coping mechanisms and strength, adversity becomes a problem when it is overwhelming and there is no foundation of resilience to overcome it. "When we talk about my neighborhood killing me, we usually talk about environmental toxins, but we are also talking about economic, social, and cultural toxins that exist in communities as a result of structural violence imposed from the outside," said Pinderhughes. One solution, then, is to build resilience into

[4] For more information on the Prevention Institute's Thrive tool, see https://www.preventioninstitute.org/tools/thrive-tool-health-resilience-vulnerable-environments (accessed September 15, 2016).

a community by creating safer public spaces through improvements in built environments, addressing housing quality and transportation, and reclaiming public spaces. This is not difficult, said Pinderhughes, but it needs the political, social, and economic will to help communities to transform their built environments in a way that strengthens their communities and allows them to sustain themselves rather than be dislocated.

Pinderhughes then described several examples of programs he believes illustrate different ways of building safer communities. San Francisco's BRIDGE affordable housing program has a trauma-informed community building component as part of its housing replacement initiative to help people stay in their rebuilt communities and thrive in healthy environments (Weinstein et al., 2014). The Taking Back Public Spaces program in New Orleans, Louisiana, and the Family Place Library in Chester, Pennsylvania, are two programs aiming to transform communities by rebuilding the social and educational structures that can support healthy family development. The Pine Ridge Reservation Stronghold Community is creating spaces such as skate parks and community gardens to serve as positive environments that meet the desires of the community and reflect Native American principles.

The people who provide these programs are attempting to establish foundations of equitable opportunity, restorative justice, healing circles, and economic empowerment to increase community wealth and resources that can resist the economic pressures that result from dislocation and gentrification, said Pinderhughes. Restorative justice, he explained, is an important model that helps change the way communities and individuals deal with conflict. In the best case scenario, restorative justice is intergenerational and reconnects people in a way that helps them understand the cost of crime and violence not just to an individual perspective, but to the whole community.

Another program he described is Roots of Success,[5] a national prison-based environmental literacy and work readiness curriculum that connects felons with the employment structure and green jobs in their communities. The YouthBuild[6] programs across the nation aim to rebuild communities by teaching construction skills to young people while rebuilding and revitalizing intergenerational social relationships.

As a final comment, Pinderhughes noted that social networks and infrastructures of social support, including culturally relevant mental health approaches, can strengthen and elevate social norms, promote healthy behaviors, and establish collaborations that promote healthy communities. Shifting and changing social norms, he said, means changing the

[5] For more information, see https://rootsofsuccess.org (accessed September 15, 2016).

[6] For more information, see https://www.youthbuild.org (accessed September 15, 2016).

narrative in violent communities by incorporating young people in the process of policy making, an approach being taken by the Teens in Action program in Louisville, Kentucky. He recommended that everyone should attend a Spoken Word event, which he called an incredibly powerful experience that illustrates how young people need to be incorporated into the process of changing the narrative on social norms in the community.

CHANGING BLIGHTED URBAN ENVIRONMENTS TO STOP GUN VIOLENCE[7]

"It has been said that the federal government has all the money, the states have all the power, but our cities have been left with all the problems," said Charles Branas as a preface to his remarks. The upside to that situation, as pointed out by Bruce Katz and Jennifer Bradley in their book *The Metropolitan Revolution* (2013), is that cities have been forced to innovate and develop new, homegrown ideas to deal with many problems, including firearm violence.

One such solution is to transform blighted and abandoned urban spaces as a strategy to provide opportunities for positive change and reduce violence. As an analogy, Branas drew on a model common in battling vector-borne infectious diseases. This model holds, for example, that if a brackish tidal pool is breeding mosquitos, filling in that pool is more likely to continue reducing the incidence of malaria long after funding ends than would expecting community members to continue regular applications of larvicide (Branas, 2010; Card, 2012). For urban firearm violence, the longer term solution would focus on remediating blighted urban environments, he explained, instead of focusing solely on victims, individuals responsible for gun violence, and weapons. Addressing blighted spaces as a solution to firearm violence is also supported by the public health impact pyramid framework offered by CDC Director Thomas Frieden (Frieden, 2010).[8] According to this framework, changing places would be a default contextual intervention that would have a larger and longer term impact on gun violence than most other approaches and would also contribute to tackling socioeconomic factors that are the greatest opportunities for high-impact changes to health problems like gun violence. "If you can positively affect a place, the thing people see every day on their way to work, school, or play, you might do it in a way that

---

[7] This section is the rapporteurs' synopsis of the presentation made by Charles Branas, professor of epidemiology and director of the Penn Injury Science Center and the Urban Health Lab at the University of Pennsylvania. The statements have not been endorsed or verified by the National Academies of Sciences, Engineering, and Medicine.

[8] To view a figure of the framework, see http://ajph.aphapublications.org/doi/pdf/10.2105/AJPH.2009.185652 (accessed September 14, 2016).

helps people and makes things better without asking them to do anything," said Branas. CDC is promoting this idea, he added, in its approach of making the healthy choice the easy choice, and it goes along with the concept that the less you ask of the people who would benefit from a program, the greater the probability of success of that program. For example, mandating that cars have airbags and changing roadways to make them safer has likely had a far more lasting and high-impact effect on reducing automobile mortality and morbidity than driver education programs.

Before discussing specific programs, Branas asked for practitioners in the field to think more about conducting randomized controlled trials and carefully designed quasi-experimental studies to learn what works. He noted that the Office of Management and Budget (OMB) issued a notice in 2013 encouraging agencies to support experimental and quasi-experimental approaches capable of distinguishing strong from weak evidence and measuring cost-effectiveness. In one example of such an approach, researchers in the Netherlands purposefully altered urban environments and observed how people in disordered neighborhoods behaved (Keizer et al., 2008). Not only did the presence of graffiti increase the amount of graffiti in the experimental neighborhoods, but it also increased the amount of littering and level of incivility in those neighborhoods.

A much larger study, called Moving to Opportunity, billed itself as a bold housing relocation experiment (Ludwig et al., 2011, 2012; Sciandra et al., 2013). This three-arm, five-city randomized trial of thousands of participants sponsored by the U.S. Department of Housing and Urban Development provided members of an experimental group with housing vouchers to move out of poverty. A comparison group of individuals were given housing vouchers to move anywhere, and a control group did not receive vouchers. "This was a landmark scientific work showing the impact of place," said Branas. The study found that the experimental and comparison groups scored higher on measures of physical health, mental health, and subjective well-being. However, Branas questioned whether it was wise to formulate policy that moves people rather than fixes the places where they already live given the expense of doing so and ethical considerations along the lines of what Pinderhughes noted when he addressed the effects of dislocation and gentrification.

A more sustainable, scalable, and well-accepted approach in communities, said Branas, involves in situ, place-based interventions. These in situ changes to places are local and conducted on a block-by-block basis right where people live. They do not involve building parks or other large public places, but rather making basic structural changes that are inexpensive, can be infused near homes and residents in the neighborhoods that most need them, and thus can be scaled throughout a city. For more than a decade, Philadelphia, for example, has been converting thousands of abandoned and blighted lots into green spaces at very low costs. These conversions take about a week to complete at about $1.25 per square foot, with maintenance costs of approximately $0.05 per square foot in each following year. Philadelphia has also been remediating abandoned buildings by simply cleaning graffiti and replacing their doors and windows at similarly low costs. Imagine, he said, how people living on these blocks feel when multiple green spaces for recreation suddenly appear, and boarded up houses disappear, on the block where they live. These changes affect how people interact with their local environments and, in essence, how they feel about themselves, said Branas.

Indeed, when Branas and his colleagues conducted a citywide study of 5,112 blighted properties—676 abandoned buildings and 4,436 vacant lots—that were fixed and compared to unfixed matched controls separated by at least one-quarter mile, they found an 8 percent drop in gun violence in the blocks with vacant lots that have been greened over the 3.5-year study (Branas et al., 2011). An economic analysis found that every dollar invested in the program returned $26 to taxpayers. Abandoned building remediation produced a larger 39 percent drop in gun violence with a return of $5 for every dollar invested (Kondo et al., 2015b). Based on these data, Branas believes these are promising approaches to reducing gun violence in cities. A study in Youngstown, Ohio, produced similar results (Kondo et al., 2015a).

Today, Branas and his colleagues are working with multiple cities to replicate both the vacant lot treatment and abandoned building remediation while at the same time conducting a multiple city–wide randomized controlled trial supported by the National Institutes of Health (NIH) to demonstrate the effectiveness of these approaches. In one study involving vacant lots, he and his collaborators fit people with heart rate monitors and GPS units and had them walk by newly greened lots and unremediated vacant lots. They found a biologically significant drop in heart rate when people walked by the newly greened lots, said Branas. Anecdotal evidence from interviews with community members also supports the efficacy of this approach, with multiple community members reporting that they avoid vacant lots and even take different routes to school or work to avoid interacting with abandoned spaces that they perceive as threatening. Blight remediation has also been shown to reduce self-reported levels of stress, although this is some of the first evidence that blight remediation may reduce biologic markers of stress (Branas et al., 2011; Garvin et al., 2012; South et al., 2015).

Blight remediation, said Branas, also can significantly reduce depression and serious mental illness, sedentary behavior, nuisance crimes, and perceptions of high crime and vandalism while significantly increasing

911 calls as community members strive to maintain the benefits of having a nicer looking neighborhood. Once you change an environment and improve it, people become invested, and that changes many of the informal policing structures that residents themselves suddenly participate in to maintain their neighborhood, explained Branas.

One interesting finding has been that firearm violence is reduced by blight remediation strategies, but other types of violence is less affected, perhaps because blighted spaces can serve as "storage lockers" for illegal guns. Early evidence from a randomized controlled trial of vacant lot greening, said Branas, showed that the magnitude of these reductions in firearm violence was most pronounced in neighborhoods below the poverty line. His team is now launching an abandoned building trial in Philadelphia, and is working with local academic partners in Flint, Michigan; Youngstown and Columbus, Ohio; Norfolk, Virginia; New Orleans, Louisiana; and both Camden and Newark, New Jersey. He also noted that the federal government has taken an interest in this approach via its Healthy People 2020 program and via support from CDC and NIH.

DISCUSSION

Richmond asked Pinderhughes and Branas for ideas on how to prevent gentrification and dislocation from happening after a community has undergone improvement. Pinderhughes responded that the places that are more successful at avoiding displacement do not make changes without community participation and without giving communities, particularly young people, real decision-making power about how these programs are implemented in their neighborhoods. Pinderhughes suggested this inclusive approach whether it involves having community members build parks and create public gardens or formulate changes in policing policies. As an example, he mentioned that Oakland, California, has instituted a police body camera policy, formulated after conversations between young people and police officers, that focuses on day-to-day interactions rather than on catching misbehavior by police officers. The goal set by these two groups was to better understand those interactions and improve them in a way that would build relationships at the community level so that police officers would be seen as members of the community. Branas stressed the importance of being ever vigilant about gentrification and forced out-migration (a key metric of gentrification) of residents from newly rehabilitated neighborhoods. One approach is to involve local, minority-owned businesses in projects that will create jobs for residents within those neighborhoods. That has been a valuable way to produce something of additional tangible value to residents and directly incorporate neighborhood voices, said Branas.

Pinderhughes added two words: anchor institutions. "Every institution represented here should take their role seriously as an anchor institution and be able to supply wealth in underserved communities," he said. Branas then asked those at the workshop from universities to be aware that many of their institutions have historically done the opposite of this. He also said that local governments need to craft policies that can try to stem gentrification, and he encouraged the workshop attendees to watch the documentary film *The Vanishing City*,[9] which explores the reasons why gentrification has happened to such a large extent in New York City and other cities like San Francisco. Philadelphia, on the other hand, has enacted policies that reduce property taxes for long-term, multigenerational residents and other mechanisms as a means of stemming gentrification (Williams, 2014). That type of action, along with rent controls, can be important tools for maintaining the diversity and economically mixed nature of many city neighborhoods, which is part of the reason people choose to live in cities in the first place, said Branas.

Terry Allan from the Cuyahoga County (Ohio) Health Department wondered if there is an opportunity to understand potential synergistic effects of multiple interventions within neighborhoods and use the resulting data to plan and fund projects that combine physical and community-based interventions. Pinderhughes responded that funding and programming are so siloed that it becomes very difficult to take a more comprehensive approach at a policy level. "I have worked with cities across the country, and it is difficult to get true collaboration across agencies that share data, information, and processes," said Pinderhughes. An additional challenge, he added, is selling at a political level the need for a longitudinal, long-term strategy. In a follow-up comment, Allan wondered if there were opportunities for key stakeholders and influencers to have an impact on the siloed funding by talking to funders and stressing the importance of integration.

Branas said he and his colleagues have worked with community groups in Youngstown, Ohio, to combine their efforts with city involvement in rehabilitating derelict spaces in the city. This effort, which he said was done with little funding, appears to have enhanced the reduction in gun violence, but further study is needed to fully understand that effect. Pinderhughes then added that HOPE SF, a project to transform San Francisco's most distressed public housing sites into thriving

[9] For more information, see http://www.thevanishingcity.com (accessed September 15, 2016).

mixed-income communities, would be a good example of a project worth examining.[10]

Jeffrey Levi of The George Washington University noted that the OMB's Office of Community Solutions is looking for opportunities to blend funding streams to make it easier to do these kinds of projects at the local level. He then offered the opinion that randomized controlled trials are not always the best methodology for use in these communities given the history of how such trials were designed unethically in the past. More importantly, he said, "The lack of funding for this kind of work over time means that if OMB wants us to wait until we have those evidence-based interventions, we are not going to be intervening in those communities for a really long time and I do not think we can afford to wait for that." Pinderhughes responded that community members in the cities he has worked with have been eager participants in designing and running experimental trials and they are greatly interested in the results of those trials. He also said that philanthropy, not government, will need to provide funding for these kinds of trials. Branas remarked that prior to producing evidence that rehabilitating empty lots and abandoned buildings actually worked, Philadelphia had smaller blight reduction programs that would come and go in a single neighborhood of the city. Only now has the city begun institutionalizing these programs on a citywide basis, informed to a generous extent by scientific studies that have emerged in recent years. Branas also noted that natural and quasi-experiments that can be done quickly and for less money can also be of great value to policy makers and help institutionalize more of these programs.

Levi then remarked that Pinderhughes and Branas addressed community trauma at the neighborhood level and noted that within neighborhoods are communities of identity, such as the LGBTQ community in Orlando, Florida. He asked what actions can be taken to address trauma at the level of communities of identity. Pinderhughes replied that as these programs spread across communities, he is seeing more interactions that perhaps can address communities of identity that do not necessarily live in the same physical community. He again reiterated the need to involve young people in whatever programs are developed and enacted.

Kahaari Kenyatta of the University of Pennsylvania asked the panelists how broadly they conceive community to be and the potential for national traumatization given the frequency of mass violence that has

[10] Anne Griffith of Enterprise Community Partners gave a presentation to the roundtable on HOPE SF. For more information, see NASEM (2016a). A video of Griffith's presentation at the June 4, 2015, workshop may also be viewed at http://www.nationalacademies.org/hmd/Activities/PublicHealth/PopulationHealthImprovementRT/2015-JUN-04/Videos/Panel%20III/17-Griffith-Video.aspx (accessed September 15, 2016).

occurred recently in this country. Pinderhughes replied that the nation is clearly traumatized, so the question becomes how to heal at the community level and then move to the societal level. "There has got to be some way in which we conceptualize the issue of healing as something we need to move through in common and incorporate into our cultural practice," said Pinderhughes. He suggested that this needs to happen in schools. A second component is getting the American public to understand how traumatized it has become and to recognize this as a problem the nation needs to address.

Samara Ford, an undergraduate at Harvard College, asked how the nature of education in the nation's schools and the ways in which students are taught or not taught about the environments in which they live interact with the bigger structural issues the speakers discussed. Branas provided one final anecdote as a response. Teachers in the Philadelphia School District are taking schoolchildren on walks through their neighborhoods and teaching them about the history of their neighborhoods and the changes that have occurred since their parents and grandparents grew up in those same neighborhoods. This program is educating children about the physical and historic contexts within which they live and asking them to think about their neighborhoods in new ways, which perhaps will instill an urge to protect and improve the places they see every day.

Pinderhughes reported that he was shocked to learn at a recent White House conference on school expulsions and suspensions that there are 10 states in which preschool children are expelled, a phenomenon that he believes is a result of the trauma these children are experiencing. "Trauma-informed pedagogy has to become part of what happens in education in inner cities and across the nation," said Pinderhughes. Some of this country's best community-based youth organizations are conducting reeducation around the dynamics of their communities, he said. The RYSE Center[11] in Richmond, California, for example, has young people think about how their community has become the way it is as a strategy to help them understand some of the dynamics of structural violence and develop the tools and foundation to become advocates and activists in their community. These types of educational programs will be needed, said Pinderhughes, to unleash the power of the nation's young people to promote change.

[11] For more information, see http://rysecenter.org (accessed September 15, 2016).

4

Local Strategies to Build Community Resilience and Safety

The workshop's second panel session featured two examples of programs building resilience and safety at the community level. Roberto Rodríguez, outreach worker supervisor for Stand Up to Violence (SUV) at Jacobi Medical Center, described the public health model he and his colleagues are using to address violence in the community. DeVone Boggan, founder and chief executive officer of Advance Peace, then discussed a program he created in Richmond, California, to address gun violence by working directly with the individuals most responsible for gun violence in that community. After the presentations, Lourdes Rodríguez, program officer at the New York State Health Foundation, moderated an open discussion. Highlights and main points made by individual speakers are in Box 4-1.

A PUBLIC HEALTH MODEL FOR TREATING VIOLENCE[1]

The Cure Violence Health Model, developed by Gary Slutkin of the University of Illinois at Chicago (Ransford et al., 2013),[2] recognizes violence as a contagious disease and a public health crisis, said Roberto

[1] This section is the rapporteurs' synopsis of the presentation made by Roberto Rodríguez, outreach worker supervisor for Stand Up to Violence (SUV) at Jacobi Medical Center. The statements have not been endorsed or verified by the National Academies of Sciences, Engineering, and Medicine.

[2] For more information on the Cure Violence Health Model, see http://cureviolence.org/the-model/essential-elements (accessed November 2, 2016).

BOX 4-1
Highlights and Main Points Made by Individual Speakers[a]

- One important role for outreach workers is to not only get violent individuals to change their behaviors and quit the lifestyle that exposes them to violence, but also change the mindset of individuals who want to join the violent gang subculture before they do (R. Rodríguez).
- A critical aspect of the Cure Violence program is that the outreach workers are always out canvassing their neighborhoods, which means that program participants do not have to go to an office or wait until the next day to talk to someone. Instead of mulling over and getting angry about a recent argument with some perceived enemy, these individuals can find their outreach workers, who can then deescalate the situation (R. Rodríguez).
- The key to stopping gun violence is to engage directly with and be informed by those individuals who are suspected to be the most lethal active firearm offenders and who have avoided sustained criminal consequences (Boggan).
- The fact that 21 of the most lethal individuals in Richmond, California, came to the Office of Neighborhood Safety in city hall to have a conversation about violence was a testament to the outreach workers, but it also showed that these young men wanted something to believe in that was designed specifically for them (Boggan).
- There must be a deliberate and intentional approach to value the assets these individuals bring to the table and to value these individuals as an important part of the solution to the problem of gun violence (Boggan).

[a] This list is the rapporteurs' summary of the main points made by individual speakers (noted in parentheses), and the statements have not been endorsed or verified by the National Academies of Sciences, Engineering, and Medicine.

Rodríguez. Slutkin noticed that similar to disease, gun violence in Chicago occurred in clusters.

Slutkin based Cure Violence on the premise that violence is a solvable contagious disease. Studies by independent external evaluators of Cure Violence programs in Chicago, Baltimore, and New York show that this idea has merit. After implementing the program, in Chicago, for example, shootings fell by 75 percent, and in Baltimore murders fell by 56 percent. Today, Cure Violence is ranked as 1 of the top 10 nongovernmental organizations in the world by the *Global Journal*, and it has been deployed in more than 23 U.S. cities and more than 50 neighborhoods in 8 countries on 5 continents, said Rodríguez.

The Cure Violence disease model has three major components. The first component aims to interrupt transmission to stop violent events before they happen, primarily by interrupting conflict to prevent retaliation. The second component involves identifying and changing the thinking of the highest potential transmitters of violence, largely those involved in the gang lifestyle, to reduce the number of violent individuals in the community. The third component works to change community norms to create social pressure to stop violence, which Rodríguez explained requires engaging community leaders, residents, business owners, and faith leaders to bring awareness to the devastation gun violence has on communities and to change attitudes so that community members reject violence in the community. Too often, he added, community members become desensitized to violence and accept it as the way things are. Overcoming that acceptance is an important step to changing community norms.

The Cure Violence program at the Jacobi Medical Center[3] covers three precincts in the northern section of the Bronx where the prevalence of gun violence has been high, and it deploys teams of credible messengers to work in the community and target those individuals who are at highest risk of committing violence. The most effective credible messengers at Jacobi are health outreach workers who live in the neighborhood and often share the same background as the highest risk individuals whom they engage, Rodríguez explained. "Outreach workers already have the trust of those high-risk individuals and therefore are more able to influence and change behavior," he said. One important role for these outreach workers is to not only get violent individuals to change their behaviors and quit the lifestyle that exposes them to violence, but also change the mindset of individuals who want to join the violent gang subculture.

The primary targets of the program are individuals who are active in a street gang, have a history of violence, are engaged in high-risk activity, and carry a weapon. Many have been shot recently or released from prison, and while the program's primary concern is to target youths between 14 and 25 years old, there are individuals older than that in the program who Rodríguez characterized as still behaving like adolescents by causing destruction in their neighborhoods, he said.

Participation in Cure Violence is completely voluntary, which is an important point, said Rodríguez, because it makes it easier for the targeted individuals to be receptive to and engage in the program. Each outreach worker has a caseload of up to 15 participants, and their role is similar to that of a social worker in that they screen, assess, and create a treatment plan designed to meet each client's needs. Perhaps 90 percent of the participants do not have jobs and are not enrolled in school, so the outreach workers help the participants find jobs, get their general edu-

[3] For more information, see https://johnjayrec.nyc/2015/04/15/suv (accessed August 23, 2016).

cational development degree, and in some cases, even help participants enroll in college. Outreach workers and other program staff even take the participants on field trips.

Rodríguez, who said he loves engaging with his clients, recounted an incident where one of his clients, out of the blue, contacted him via Facetime. His client held out his hand and showed him bullets. Instead of trying to counsel him via phone or put him down, Rodríguez said he shifted the conversation by blaming himself for failing his client. Several days later, his client came up to him and apologized and shared that he had a falling out with his mother. "Sometimes these youth are crying out for help, but they do not like to disclose what they might be going through in their lives," said Rodríguez. "A lot of them are guarded and resistant toward seeking any type of treatment." A critical aspect of the program is that the outreach workers are always out canvassing their neighborhoods, which means that program participants do not have to go to an office or wait until the next day to talk to someone. Instead of mulling over and getting angry about a recent argument with some perceived enemy, these individuals can find their outreach workers, who can then deescalate the situation.

To illustrate Cure Violence's power to prevent violence, Rodríguez discussed one of the major conflicts in the Jacobi program's target area. Two gangs, New Jack and Fever Block, had been engaged in an ongoing conflict, so the program conducted a formal mediation in the office on two consecutive days. Those sessions identified a Fever Block member as a good candidate to be an outreach worker, and in fact, the program hired him and he has become very influential in the two neighborhoods in which these gangs are active. Though still active, there have been no shootings between these two gangs, and they have even come together without conflict at multiple events.

The program treats violence as a community health problem, so it is imperative to engage the community as a whole, explained Rodríguez. This occurs on a daily basis as the caseworkers canvas their neighborhoods and interact with community residents. Program employees participate in shooting responses organized by clergy leaders, elected officials, and friends and family of the victims to help mobilize the community to partake in peaceful antiviolence marches 72 hours after a shooting. "It could be a stabbing, but we focus on shootings because our mission is to try to prevent gun violence in the community," explained Rodríguez.

Over the 2 years the program at Jacobi has been operating, gun violence in the target area has fallen by 53 percent. An advantage of running this program out of a hospital is that it creates an opportunity to bridge the gap between the health system and the community. The Jacobi Medical Center is the primary trauma center facility in the Bronx, so all shooting victims are taken there, giving the program's hospital-based responders the opportunity to engage a victim in the emergency department and take steps to prevent retaliation. "There is someone by their bedside trying to engage them, something a social worker is unable to do," said Rodríguez. The hospital-based responders are people who victims can identify with and relate to, so they are less guarded and may be more responsive to probing and provide information to the responders that may help prevent a violent retaliation.

The hospital also plays a role in the program once the patient is discharged, said Rodríguez. A team consisting of a social worker, pediatrician, and hospital responder sees the patient on a weekly basis. At the same time, a pastor and outreach worker get involved on a more constant basis to serve as mentors who can guide the individual through a difficult time. The hospital also serves as the nexus for follow-on support in the form of specialized social, educational, vocational, and recreational services.

AN INCLUSIVE APPROACH TO ADVANCING PEACE[4]

For DeVone Boggan, the key to stopping gun violence is to engage directly with and be informed by those individuals who are suspected to be the most lethal, active firearm offenders and who have avoided sustained criminal consequences. It is important to understand that one's journey to becoming a serial shooter occurs because less than 30 percent of shooters in most urban communities are ever prosecuted for their gun crimes, said Boggan. The message that statistic sends, he explained, is that the formal justice system does not work in those communities, that shooters can act with impunity, and that victims and their associates will find their own way to get justice, which often can involve becoming a shooter, too.

Any solution to this problem, said Boggan, should include and be informed by the people at the center of firearm conflict. The challenge, then, is to find, engage, and meet these people where they are in their development. Making this challenge more difficult, he said, is the fact that the experiences these individuals have had with people like him is that they come with empty promises and unrealistic expectations. We have to be willing to authentically engage these individuals in a respectful manner in spite of what they have allegedly done or are suspected of doing, in spite of the fact that he may have seven casualties on his belt,

[4] This section is the rapporteurs' synopsis of the presentation made by DeVone Boggan, founder and chief executive officer of Advance Peace. The statements have not been endorsed or verified by the National Academies of Sciences, Engineering, and Medicine.

said Boggan. In doing so, he added, it is important to understand that these young men are isolated and alone, negotiating all kinds of direct and vicarious untreated traumas, and they are enraged. Accepting these young people as partners and as a significant part of the solution to reducing gun violence is a key step for success, he added, while acknowledging how hard that can be. These are our most difficult and challenging young people, he said, but we must see their inherent value and humanity. Only then can we embrace them.

For more than 8 years, Boggan was the neighborhood safety director for the City of Richmond, California's Office of Neighborhood Safety. Richmond, located 17 miles northeast of San Francisco, has a diverse population of approximately 100,000 and has historically had a gun violence problem. Over a 20-year period from 1986 to 2005, nearly 700 people were murdered, an average of almost 35 per year. In 2006, Boggan recounted, the number of people killed by gunfire jumped to 42, and then to 47 in 2007 and 47 again in 2008. In Richmond, young men and women who are engaged in firearm activity come from an environment in which there have been generations of gun-related hostilities and where more often than not they have fathers, uncles, cousins, and friends who have been affected by gun violence. For the young men in North Richmond and Central Richmond, the feeling is that someone from the other side of town is responsible for a terrorist attack against them and they grow up believing it is their responsibility to bring justice to the enemy, year after year after year, generation after generation after generation, said Boggan.

In 2007, Boggan was hired as the founding director of the newly created Office of Neighborhood Safety. This non–law enforcement agency was formed to specifically address gun violence, rather than gang violence in general, and to be responsible for capacity building to support the reduction of gun violence and improve coordination of services across government and nongovernmental institutions in this area. The creation of this office was a big step, said Boggan, because gang violence prevention programs rarely focus on active firearm offenders. In fact, he added, most gang members do not become shooters, and neither do most people released from prison.

Given the authority to go directly to the individuals most responsible for gun violence, Boggan began hiring ex-felons with a gun-related crime on their record as full-time city employees. These individuals would be his program's credible messengers. Although many people thought this was a strange idea, Boggan noted that the four individuals he hired in 2008 to be neighborhood change agents are still with the program today, which he said has led to increased trust on the streets between the city agency workers and the people they engage. This stability has been vital to their success. "It is not a revolving door as it relates to engaging this population and better appreciating and understanding why they shoot and what is going to be required for them to not shoot to address conflict," he explained.

From 2008 to 2009, Boggan and his four colleagues engaged in a broad and generalized street, community, and school outreach program that was very intentional in its efforts to identify those individuals who were most responsible for gun violence in the community. In discussions with local, state, and federal law enforcement officials working on gun crimes, Boggan learned that 28 people were thought to be responsible for 70 percent of the 45 gun-related murders and 186 non-fatal shootings in 2009. Astonished by the fact that 28 people were largely responsible for the gun violence in these communities, Boggan met with his outreach workers and told them that these 28 individuals would be the focus of his office's efforts for the next year. "No more broad, hot-spot outreach activity," said Boggan. "We were going to do hot-people engagement activity. Why hot people? Because hot spots are dictated by hot people," and hot people can and do move. He gave his outreach workers 3 months to convince these 28 people to come to city hall to talk to him, to ensure them that this was not a sophisticated law enforcement sting, and that he had an alternative lifestyle opportunity he wanted to present to them.

In June 2010, the Operation Peacemaker Fellowship was started with the 21 young men—3 were lost to gunfire and 4 did not choose to participate—who arrived at city hall in three groups to discuss how they could partner with Boggan and his staff to reduce gun violence in Richmond. That 21 of the most lethal individuals in Richmond came to city hall was a testament to the outreach workers, but it also showed that these young men wanted something to believe in that was designed specifically for them. What the men got, said Boggan, was the offer to accept a non-mandated, high-touch graduate school–like Fellowship with six components. First, they would receive multiple contacts every day from several healthy people. Second, Boggan promised to sit down with each Fellow and create a life map with smart goals for the 18 months of the Fellowship and the opportunities that meeting those goals would afford them. Third, they would be connected with every social service opportunity, and not just by pointing them in the right direction, but actually taking them to appointments and making sure they get the best services available.

Fourth, the Fellowships came with a stipend of $9,000 over 18 months, and although the media liked to portray this as paying criminals to stop shooting, Boggan said he never asks these young men to stop shooting or even put down their guns. "Why not?" he asked. Boggan and his colleagues did not want their privileged perspective and position to render them non-credible, he explained. The Fellows live in war zones, and for them it is a rational idea to carry a gun. Boggan added that $9,000 is a small amount of money for the city to pay men who are partnering with the city to reduce gun violence, particularly when compared to the high costs that accrue each time a young man is shot.[5]

The goal of this high-touch approach, he said, is to reduce shootings and to bring these young men into the mainstream so they can have meaningful opportunities to engage in the community, and so the program's fifth component is to provide what the Fellows have told Boggan are transformative life excursions. In California, these young men can travel throughout the state with Boggan and other Fellows. They visit universities, talk to officials in the cities they visit, do community service activities they cannot do at home because of safety reasons, and above all, they have fun. "It is amazing when you take a 27-year-old young man to Disneyland and at the end of the day he walks up to you with Mickey Mouse ears on and he says, 'Boss man,' with tears in his eyes, 'that's one of the best experiences I've ever had,'" said Boggan.

The Fellows also get to travel out of the state and even out of the country, but for that opportunity the Fellows must be willing to travel with someone they are suspected of trying to kill and who allegedly has been trying to kill them. "It is an amazing experience to show up on Robben Island in South Africa with groups of men who have been trying to take each other's lives for the last 3 to 5 years and they come to a common understanding," and a new respect for one another, "not a Kumbaya experience," said Boggan.

The sixth component puts a council of elders around each of these individuals, men who have retired or are near retirement and who have had successful careers and have successful, healthy families. Howard Pinderhughes (see Chapter 3), Boggan noted, is one of the men who works with his program. What is important is that these elders are not afraid of these young men and are willing to talk to them and meet them where they are, said Boggan.

After 18 months in the program, most of these men are not the same people they were when they showed up at city hall to hear the Fellowship offer. They have a better appreciation for authority and for showing up for work every day. Equally important, said Boggan, "We have a better understanding of who they are and what their interests and passions are." Using that knowledge, he is better able to connect these young men to subsidized internships that they might actually want to stay in rather than getting them a job merely to have a job. Today, of the three cohorts

[5] According to the California Legislative Analyst's Office, the cost of incarcerating an individual in 2008–2009 in California was $47,102 per year. See http://www.lao.ca.gov/PolicyAreas/CJ/6_cj_inmatecost (accessed September 9, 2016).

that have finished the program and the fourth that is now enrolled, 94 percent of individuals—the most lethal active firearm offenders who are also the most likely to be victims of gunfire—are alive 2 to 5 years out, and 84 percent have not been injured by a firearm since becoming a Fellow. Perhaps more importantly, said Boggan, 79 percent of the Fellows have not become a suspect in a new firearm crime based on local and regional law informant intelligence. The bottom line, he said, is that these numbers translate into lives saved, as evidenced by a 75 percent reduction in firearm-related murders and a 66 percent reduction in firearm assaults with an injury between 2007 and 2015.

The take-home lesson, he said in closing, is that our most effective efforts to reduce urban gun violence must be comprehensive, developmental, and informed by the young men at the center of firearm conflict. "Only then [will our efforts be truly] credible and legitimate from their vantage point, and only then can it truly be responsive to who these young men are and what these young men have experienced," said Boggan.

DISCUSSION

Lourdes Rodríguez began the discussion by commenting that the programs the two speakers described offer the potential to redefine where society invests its money—in programs that turn felons into Fellows, or in so-called million-dollar blocks,[6] where millions of dollars are spent incarcerating people who live on particular streets. She then asked the panelists to comment on how they look past the problematic behaviors these individuals might have to see their aspirations and how their life experiences could lead to change. Boggan said there has to be a deliberate and intentional approach to value the assets these individuals bring to the table and to value these individuals as an important part of the solution to the problem of gun violence. He recounted how when he brought the first group of young men to city hall, he provided name tags with their legal names, not street names, informational Fellowship packets in front of their placards, and lots of good food. He then apologized on behalf of the city for taking so long to ask them to get involved in solving a problem that clearly required their help, experience, and expertise. On behalf of the city, Boggan was asking them to be partners in the effort to stop gun violence in Richmond. "How I, as the neighborhood safety director, communicated that day meant something, and that is why every one of the 21 young men who showed up said they wanted to be part of this team." He noted that an evaluation of the program showed how the attitudes of

[6] For more information, see http://www.npr.org/2012/10/02/162149431/million-dollar-blocks-map-incarcerations-costs (accessed August 31, 2016).

these young men changed because of their involvement—they saw the Office of Neighborhood Safety as family.

Roberto Rodríguez agreed that these young men are the agents of change and that the key rests in three words: self-esteem, empowerment, and optimism. "When you believe in folks who are prone to violence, prone to doing wrong, prone to negativity, it sends a strong message," said Rodríguez. "It gives them a sense of hope." He also said he knows this from his own personal experience, that having individuals believe in him is what enabled him to transform his life after spending 16 years in prison. "I believe that when you steer someone in the right direction genuinely, you will see good results."

Catherine Baase of The Dow Chemical Company asked Boggan how to move upstream from the type of work he is doing, that is, how to intervene before individuals are past the point of transformation. Boggan responded that it is important to recognize how engaging these young men developmentally can work for the community as compared to broad law enforcement raids that pull them into the criminal justice system. "If we are able to successfully develop these young men, in spite of what they are suspected of doing, versus pulling them temporarily into the criminal justice system, what we are able to do is to begin to slowly change the dynamics of what is going on in that very community." He noted that when law enforcement pulls these individuals out of the community, they are rapidly replaced by others or people simply wait for their return and the continuation of business as usual. By contrast, keeping the young men who are not charged or convicted in the community and turning them into change agents can stop that cycle and change behavior in the next generation of potential shooters.

These actions alone will not be enough, he added. He suggested that the current social services platform could be retooled to make it more outreach oriented so that staff people are going into the communities to reach young people standing on the corner rather than waiting for them to come to the community center for help. Boggan added that unless the mainstream social service and public health platforms are pushed to intentionally engage in the areas of a community where gun violence is concentrated where many young "upstream" individuals exist, but are rarely if ever touched by the current platforms, he will never be put out of business, which is his ultimate goal.

Daniel Webster of the Johns Hopkins Bloomberg School of Public Health noted that he has been studying how to prevent violence for about 25 years and what Boggan shared at the workshop is consistent with everything that he has learned. He then asked for ideas on how to engage these young men, many of whom want to kill one another, to get past the idea of retaliation and payback that is behind so much urban gun violence. Rodríguez replied that an approach his program has taken is to get these individuals together out of their comfort zones and expose them to a different environment, which enables these individuals to see each other in a new light and get them talking to one another as two humans rather than two adversaries. These interactions, said Rodríguez, can change the entire dynamics of their relationships. He recounted how one of his outreach workers, who had been a member of the Bloods, would not travel to an area considered Crips territory because he feared for his safety. However, when the program hired a Crips member from that area to be an outreach worker, the two ended up bonding and creating a relationship that is now changing the norms in their two communities.

Both Rodríguez and Boggan said that such a transformation is a process, not something that happens overnight. That process, explained Boggan, aims to take these individuals from a place where they do not care about the future to one where they do, from one where they feel alone to one where they feel loved and accounted for, which is new to them. Once these individuals start caring, they start reconsidering their decisions about how to negotiate conflict.

Boggan noted that nobody in his program can fail their Fellowship, even if they shoot someone during the 18-month program. Fellows can leave voluntarily or if they are taken into custody by law enforcement and convicted of committing a crime, they forfeit their Fellowship opportunity. "The Fellowship is designed for an active firearm offender, so why punish him for doing something that we know he does?" asked Boggan. The important thing, he said, is to continue to love these young men and to leverage every opportunity to continue to support these young men through the process of changing their mindsets. He added that every time he travels out of state, he brings several of these young men with him, often accompanied by his wife and children.

Sanne Magnan commented that what she heard from the two speakers and their stories is the importance of engagement, respect, building trust, and humility in keeping these young men alive. What she wanted to know, though, is what the narrative has to be with their bosses to keep these programs alive. Boggan said that in Richmond it has taken a great deal of effort as well as a very supportive city manager in addition to statistics that demonstrate the program's success. He added that it is hard work and a challenging process because many people do not understand these young men. People are afraid of them and what they may attract to the organizational environment and therefore resist and neglect working to support their development. Boggan noted that the first thing to get cut when budgets are tight are these types of programs, despite their proven success, when in his opinion cities and investment partners such as philanthropy need to double down on their investment in these efforts. He added that strong philanthropic support is important too, both in terms of financial support, but also in sending the message that these programs have to survive and remain a viable part of city government funding portfolios if further philanthropic resources are going to be committed and sustained.

Rodríguez commented that these young men are faced with a double-edged sword in that their reputations in their communities are what enable them to be credible messengers who are relevant in those communities, and yet they also need to move away from the behaviors that built those reputations. He also said that safety is a concern for him and his teams when they are out canvassing their neighborhoods. However, the outreach workers have learned when confronted by old adversaries how to make better judgments, and Rodríguez expressed confidence in their ability to diffuse a volatile situation without violence.

Maria Santiago of the Healing Center asked if these programs include discussions about partner violence and the roles men need to play in the lives of their partners and children. Rodríguez said Cure Violence's treatment plans include peer-to-peer counseling and access to resources on parenting, substance abuse, and other subjects that can increase the vulnerability of these young men. He noted how important it is for these young men to identify with peers who have changed their lives because too many of them do not know how to ask for help. Boggan added that it is important to address all of the issues that impact young men, which includes family, parenting, and being a good partner.

5

Lessons Learned: Evaluating Community- and Hospital-Based Models and Initiatives

The workshop's third set of presentations examined some of the lessons learned from programs directed at curbing violence. Daniel Webster, professor of health and policy management at the Johns Hopkins Bloomberg School of Public Health, director of the Johns Hopkins Center for Gun Policy and Research, and deputy director for research for the Johns Hopkins Center for the Prevention of Youth Violence, first described the influence of Baltimore's Safe Streets Program. Jeffrey Butts, director of the Research and Evaluation Center at John Jay College of Criminal Justice, then reviewed his research team's evaluation of New York's Cure Violence program, and Thea James, vice president of mission and associate chief medical officer at the Boston Medical Center, discussed the implementation and expansion of a hospital-based violence intervention advocacy program. Following the three presentations, Webster moderated an open discussion among the workshop participants. Highlights and main points made by individual speakers are in Box 5-1.

LESSONS LEARNED FROM BALTIMORE'S SAFE STREETS PROGRAM[1]

When Webster began working in Baltimore nearly 25 years ago, the city already had a long history with gun violence. In 2006, after Webster

[1] This section is the rapporteurs' synopsis of the presentations made by Daniel Webster, professor of health and policy management at the Johns Hopkins Bloomberg School of Pub-

BOX 5-1
Highlights and Main Points Made by Individual Speakers[a]

- In talking about evidence-based programs, whether it be Cure Violence or a focused deterrence approach, implementation matters, as does who is involved in carrying out an intervention (Webster).
- When it comes to measuring violence, there is no such thing as data on the incidence of violence, but rather data on proxies of violence, such as injuries reported by hospitals or police reports (Butts).
- If experimental design is treated as the only evidence that can be used to evaluate program effectiveness, then the only studies done to shape policy that focus on changing behavior will focus on the individual rather than community level (Butts).
- Helping individuals to leverage their own personal strengths and assets can affect population health and even prevention when dealing with a young person who has children. Doing so can be a form of treatment, and it can break cycles of violence (James).
- The most important element of the Violence Intervention Advocacy Program is that it provides young individuals with one caring adult on whom they can depend and trust (James).
- It is important to respect the workers that make or break these programs and to pay them commensurate with the dangerous work they are expected to do in their communities (Butts, Webster).
- The real value of these program models is the fact that there are people from a neighborhood with the background and experience to be credible messengers and they have the ability to tap into the information available in the community about the conflicts that are about to erupt (Butts).

[a] This list is the rapporteurs' summary of the main points made by individual speakers (noted in parentheses), and the statements have not been endorsed or verified by the National Academies of Sciences, Engineering, and Medicine.

and his colleagues returned from a visit to Chicago to learn more about Cure Violence (then known as Ceasefire), the city decided to try the program, and he has been involved in evaluating this program since then.

On a staggered schedule, from July 2007 to November 2008, the city started the Safe Streets Baltimore program in five neighborhoods, with two still in operation. One of these neighborhoods, known as Cherry Hill, is geographically isolated from the rest of the city, noted Webster. More recently, the city introduced the program in a west Baltimore neighbor-

lic Health, director of the Johns Hopkins Center for Gun Policy and Research, and deputy director for research for the Johns Hopkins Center for the Prevention of Youth Violence. The statements have not been endorsed or verified by the National Academies of Sciences, Engineering, and Medicine.

hood, Mondawmin, which is where the uprising began after Freddie Gray's death; in the neighboring Sandtown area; and in the northwest Baltimore neighborhood called Lower Park Heights.

To assess how the Safe Streets program affected attitudes, Webster and his colleagues developed and validated a tool that uses common scenarios that lead to shootings based on research and information obtained from Baltimore's youth (see Table 5-1). He noted that the neighborhoods had similar risk factors that could be easily assessed in a short on-street survey, and that after controlling for individual-level risk facts, there was a "fairly powerful deterrent effect" with regard to changing attitudes about the acceptability of using guns to resolve conflicts in a variety of circumstances (Milam et al., 2016).

The influence of the program on homicides and shootings was mixed. By May 2012, two of the neighborhoods experienced a drop in homicides, 21 percent in McElderry Park and 34 percent in Cherry Hill, but in one neighborhood, Madison East End, where the program had been running for only 18 months, the homicide rate rose by 200 percent. That is a relatively rare outcome, but that is what they found. Webster noted that non-fatal shootings fell by 41 percent in Madison East End and 34 percent in Elwood Park. In some but not all neighborhoods, there was a spillover effect in that violence decreased in surrounding neighborhoods. One interesting finding, said Webster, was that outreach workers of the type Roberto Rodríguez of Stand Up to Violence described in Chapter 4 were

TABLE 5-1 Attitudinal Question on the Legitimacy of Using Guns to Settle Disputes

Do you think it's okay to shoot/ threaten someone with a gun when...	Yes	No	Maybe
I am at a club with my girl and this guy is dancing with her.			
I see a guy on the street who beat up my brother last week.			
I see a guy on the street who robbed me of $50 and my Timberland boots.			
I see a guy who has not paid me the $100 he owes me.			
A guy disrespects me on the street in front of my friends. I think the guy is carrying a gun.			

SOURCE: Webster presentation, June 16, 2016.

having the same effect at reducing gun violence as was a focused deterrence approach used by law enforcement specifically targeting offenders.

His team's most recent analysis, through December 2015, found that when aggregated across neighborhoods and duration, there was no net change in homicides associated with the program, but there was a 27 percent reduction in non-fatal shootings. The most impressive results, said Webster, occurred in the geographically isolated Cherry Hill neighborhood, where there was a 44 percent reduction in homicides and a 41 percent drop in non-fatal shootings over a 7-year span starting in November 2008 even though the resources allocated to that neighborhood were reduced. Two other neighborhoods, Lower Park Heights and McElderry Park, also saw a reduction in homicides, 38 percent and 23 percent, respectively, though the program's inability to reduce gun violence in the Mondawmin neighborhood is of great concern, said Webster. Nonetheless, he believes this program has been the most effective action Baltimore has taken to combat gun violence, even though it has only been introduced in a handful of communities. "If you look at all of the investment in a variety of different law enforcement approaches, including focused deterrence, Safe Streets has done better," said Webster. In fact, the focused deterrence model has so far not been effective in Baltimore and has been associated with more shootings.

In talking about evidence-based programs, whether Cure Violence or a focused deterrence approach, Webster believes that implementation matters, as does who is involved in carrying out an intervention. "When I think about what might explain some of the varied effects that we are seeing with this program, I mention neighborhood as being important in and of itself," said Webster. "I also think there is this aspect that is very hard to quantify in a scientific way, but it is getting the right people who can do this most challenging work."

EVALUATING THE CURE VIOLENCE PROGRAM

Before beginning their outside evaluation of the Cure Violence program, Jeffrey Butts and his colleagues collaborated with Gary Slutkin and his team at the Cure Violence headquarters in Chicago to develop a fair description of the program's model in order to lay the groundwork for a controlled study to measure the program's effectiveness. It was during this process that Butts noticed that Cure Violence's approach to attitudinal changes is to work on multiple angles simultaneously, rather than just targeting the people involved in violence and forcing them to stop.

Given the importance of norm change, Butt's team decided to measure that as well as collecting administrative data about violence in the test communities. Using and adapting some of Webster's measures, crews of young people with iPads went into the neighborhoods and conducted respondent-driven sampling. Although this survey technique has drawbacks with regard to the validity of the sample, said Butts, it is a good way to get a quick sample of the traditionally hard-to-reach and hard-to-recruit population of 18- to 30-year-old males. He explained that this was not a follow-up longitudinal panel study in which his team would go back and find the same people over time. "What we are doing is measuring the prevalent social attitudes among 18- to 30-year-old men in these neighborhoods and seeing if the trajectory of those norms about violence moves in a neighborhood that has Cure Violence versus one that does not," said Butts.

One surprise, he said, was that 40 to 50 percent of the young men surveyed in some of these neighborhoods reported they had been shot at, which could mean they were standing on a corner and someone fired a gun, and that some 20 percent had been stabbed. Unsurprising was the lack of confidence among these young men in public institutions and their ability to help the neighborhood in response to violence. Police and public officials received low marks while fire and ambulance crews received more positive reviews.

When it came to measuring violence, Butts said there is no such thing as data on the incidence of violence, but rather data on proxies of violence, such as injuries reported by hospitals. In New York City, there is a dataset available containing diagnostic codes for everyone treated in the emergency department of every hospital in the city, and that is one of the sources of outcomes data that his team has been following over time. That dataset, though, does not include all crime because in many of these neighborhoods, crime-related injuries are treated at home. Another incomplete proxy is reported crime by mid-block coordinates for shots fired, assaults, robberies with a weapon, and homicides. Butts and his team are now examining the datasets, which cover 20 years, to determine if there are changes in incidents of violence that can be associated with changes in community norms.

As a short aside, Butts challenged the research community to stop arguing about whether focusing on hot spots or hot people is the better approach. "Obviously, you have to do both," said Butts, using influenza as an analogy. "We would not say we would combat a flu epidemic just by finding the people with the flu. We would also try to teach people about how to avoid the flu." He added that while supporters of both views are good at "cherry picking" data to defend their particular approach, the reality is that solving the problem of community violence will require all of the tools at society's disposal. The key is developing the evidence to show that a given intervention is truly correlated with the cause of violence in a way that is reliable and replicable.

Butts cautioned that the demand for specific experimental designs as the only acceptable evidence for public policy excludes any model that is not delivered at the individual level. He added that no organization has the resources to do that type of study. If experimental design is treated as the only evidence that can be used to evaluate program effectiveness, then the only studies done to shape policy that focus on changing behavior will focus on the individual rather than community level. "That can work and is definitely part of the toolbox, but unless we focus on the structural and social context of all of those individual behaviors, we will not really solve this problem. We have to accept evidence that is not just experimental," said Butts.

A HOSPITAL-BASED APPROACH TO VIOLENCE INTERVENTION[2]

For Thea James, the emergency department is an ideal place to capture a young person's attention and begin to break the cycle of community violence. In the United States, more than 700,000 young people ages 12 to 24 are seen in emergency departments for non-fatal injuries sustained from assaults. Moreover, said James, up to 40 percent of young people under age 24 who are admitted for violent injuries are readmitted for subsequent violence-related injuries, and half of these youth who return are homicide victims. Violence, she added, is the leading cause of death for African American males ages 15 to 34, the second leading cause of death for young Latinos, and the fifth leading cause of death among white males in the same age group.

As a reminder to the workshop attendees, James defined the social determinants of health as the economic and social conditions that influence individual and group differences in health status as well as opportunities for employment, to get a good education, and in general to thrive (see Figure 5-1). She noted that if the cycle of violence is not broken when treating young people, who often have their own children, what happens to these young individuals is likely to happen to their children, too. In fact, she said, when she and her colleagues created Boston Medical Center's Violence Intervention Advocacy Program (VIAP),[3] which is part of the National Network of Hospital-Based Violence Intervention Programs,[4]

---

[2] This section is the rapporteurs' synopsis of the presentation made by Thea James, vice president of mission and associate chief medical officer at Boston Medical Center, and the statements have not been endorsed or verified by the National Academies of Sciences, Engineering, and Medicine.

[3] For more information, see http://www.bphc.org/whatwedo/violence-prevention/violence-intervention-advocate-program/Pages/default.aspx (accessed August 21, 2016).

[4] For more information, see http://nnhvip.org (accessed August 21, 2016).

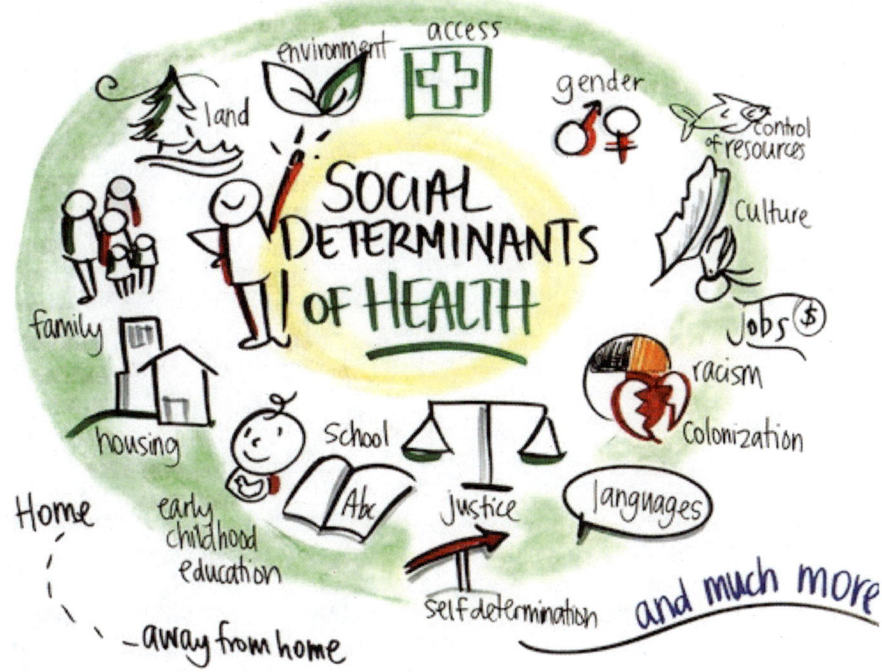

FIGURE 5-1 Social determinants of health.
SOURCE: James presentation, June 16, 2016.

they created it to provide services for both the injured individuals and their families.

Helping individuals to leverage their own personal strengths and assets can affect population health and even prevention when dealing with a young person who has children, said James. Doing so can be a form of treatment, and it can break cycles of violence, she said. "I think many people have many innate talents and strengths," said James. "They just need an opportunity to make those things come to fruition." She noted that many of the young individuals who have received the hospital-based intervention have told her that without that intervention, the cycle of violence would have continued and they would either be dead or in jail.

When James and her colleagues created VIAP, one of its main tenets was that they would do everything possible to see every young person who came to the Boston Medical Center emergency department who had been shot or stabbed. "There was no cherry picking involved," said James. "It took a while in the beginning to get the program to the point where everyone understood that the goal was to connect with every single person who come through the door. We did not have a precedent for how this works."

When developing the program, James started with the formula that parents use to help their children grow up to have opportunities for a good life. Parents make sure that they mentor their children and are there when their children need them. Parents give their children shelter, food, and opportunities for education. Parents teach their children how to navigate life, how to hold down a job, and how to be responsible. "I thought, that is what we will do. Our staff will be mentors, and we will partner with community-based organizations to provide the other specific things that people need," said James. She also accepted that because VIAP's clients are young people, these individuals would have some missteps, but just as a good parent will do, she and her team would give them the support they need to get through these challenges.

The program she and her colleague developed uses a trauma-informed approach and assumes these young individuals have experienced traumas that have shaped the way they think, their expectations, and their perspectives. Operating from that viewpoint allows staff to see many of the behaviors of these young people as manifestations of trauma rather than stubbornness at not wanting to engage in physical therapy or being surly or uncooperative when they act like they do not care about getting help. "I think any of us who had been in any way assaulted would probably react the same way," said James.

VIAP was started with five goals:

1. Provide opportunities for progress and "real" change that would put the individual on a different track in life.
2. Prevent retaliation.
3. Serve as positive role models and promote positive alternatives to violence.
4. Strengthen family networks.
5. Contribute to safer, healthier communities.

James and her team learned early that it was important to reach out to other staff to get them on board with what they were doing and gain allies among hospital staff, particularly given that the program involves staff from a wide range of departments. Outreach to other hospital staff is not something that they did in the beginning, and it caused some tension with other staff who were concerned that their roles in the hospital were being usurped. Once her team had formed alliances throughout the hospital, the program ran smoothly. Another early approach James and her colleagues used was to plot a four-stage path that these young individuals would take through the program. Stage 1 starts at intake and involves building trust and creating a relationship with an individual. There is daily contact through this stage and staff work with the individual to create a safety plan and an assessment of that individual's needs, and to complete any relevant documents. In the second stage, the program connects the individual with needed services, including transitional assistance, victim's assistance, housing, medical follow-up, primary care, and mental health counseling. Stage 3 helps the individual with personal development by connecting them with the educational system, job readiness and training programs, job opportunities, and continuing mental health services. The final stage aims to help the individual be independent and maintain the gains they have made so far while nurturing further growth and development. These stages are not set in stone, but rather serve as a means of organizing tiers of service that meet these young individuals where they are in their lives.

When the program was launched, James hired two young people from the community to be what she calls advocates and some of her colleagues call intervention specialists. These two young men worked 7 days per week from 4 p.m. to midnight, and over the course of those 8 hours they would go from room to room getting to know who these young people were, gaining an understanding of how they ended up being shot or stabbed, and developing a list of what their needs would be going forward and which partners the program would have to involve to meet those needs. These interactions, said James, gave her and her colleagues the opportunity to establish what resources the program would need to succeed, develop, and move forward. One thing they learned in this first year was that the tattoos on these young individuals were sources of information about the lives they were leading. One tattoo said, for example, "Born to be hated. Dying to be loved." Another said, "I am a product of my adversity." A third read, "Death is nothing, but to live defeated is to die every day." What these tattoos said to her, James recounted, was how hopeless these young men are, that from their perspective the trajectories of their lives were bleak and therefore they had nothing to lose. "It gave us some idea about what they would need from us from the perspective of mentorship and partnership," said James.

To James, the most important element of VIAP is having one caring adult these young individuals can depend on and trust. "That is the person who gets them on the other side of the bridge," said James. Based on their experiences in the first year, she and her colleagues have transitioned the program from being purely peer based and hospital based to a full case management model with community partnerships. The program now has three advocates serving as case managers as well as a family support coordinator, a data research manager, and an employment readiness specialist. Emergency medicine residents can now choose the program as an elective rotation, and the program also has social work interns. The program has two City street workers from Boston Centers for Youth and Families who James explained are essentially on duty in the neighborhoods 24 hours per day, 365 days per year. Every time someone gets injured or fatally wounded, these individuals receive cell phone notification texts. They go to the hospital and the bedsides of these young men and women, some of whom they have formed relationships with in the community. These street workers have proven invaluable to the families of those involved, the hospital staff, and the public safety staff. "They will often mitigate chaos in the hospital because when someone gets injured, many people from the community convene on the hospital," said James. Having the street workers at the injured individual's bedside almost immediately is invaluable, she added, because their trusted status enables them to defuse the call for retaliation.

James and her colleagues also work in tandem with a behavioral health team called the Community Violence Response Team based in the hospital's trauma department. Every person on the hospital's "protected list," which restricts visitors to protect an injured person's safety, is assigned to one of VIAP's advocates and to a member of the Community Violence Response Team. In addition, individuals can also be assigned to a family support coordinator, creating a team of three individuals looking out for each patient. This team works in tandem with victims of violence. Participation in the program is voluntary, said James, and individuals who turn down the offer to join when they are in the hospital can always join the program later.

Today, the program has a van provided by the hospital to transport program participants and move them into their new apartments, which they can live in rent free for 1 year if they have secured a job and are actively engaged in the mental health portion of the program. The program provides the participants with clothing so they make a good impression when interviewing for jobs and they get help obtaining their driver's licenses.

As a final note, James explained that program staff members serve as mentors to the advocates and street workers, as well as to their families. "We send them to many different types of training and we help them get into college." She recounted stories of one advocate who had been performing poorly in school who is now consistently an honor roll student in college and planning to go to graduate school. Another young man who had not graduated high school when he became an advocate recently invited James to come to the graduation ceremony for his M.B.A. degree.

DISCUSSION

Daniel Webster started the discussion by asking James if VIAP clients undergo formal screening for PTSD. She replied that the Community Violence Response Team does the PTSD screen. Webster also asked James to elaborate further on the trauma-informed approach her program takes. James said her staff conducts simulations in a simulation laboratory for nurses so they understand how a patient's behaviors can be manifestations of the trauma that patient has suffered. She noted as an example that after the Boston Marathon bombing, nurses reported that some patients had repeated outbursts, but nobody saw this as a negative behavior; they understood the role of trauma in the patients' actions.

Pamela Russo of the Robert Wood Johnson Foundation (RWJF) asked Webster to comment on why he thought some neighborhoods that implemented Safe Streets initiatives had better results than others. Webster replied that the neighborhoods in which the program worked best were those in which the outreach workers saw the role as a life mission. In contrast, neighborhoods that did not have good outcomes were staffed by outreach workers who saw their job as merely a means to a paycheck. "I believe that this is a program model that is highly dependent on these credible messengers building trust. Yes, they all get the same training that I am sure is helpful, but I think people bring different things to this job," said Webster. Another factor, he added, is the differences in the neighborhoods themselves. The two areas in Baltimore where the program has been least successful, he said, are the most challenged in terms of community organization and participation and the number of abandoned buildings, for example.

He also noted that this work is incredibly difficult and experience leads him to believe that the program has underinvested in its outreach workers. In fact, he added, the thing that he is least proud of with the Safe Streets program is that the salary for doing this dangerous job did not increase from 2007 to 2015. Referring back to DeVone Boggan's comments about respect (see Chapter 4), Webster emphasized that it is important to respect the workers that make or break these programs.

The real value of these models, said Butts, is the fact that you can have people from a neighborhood with the background and experience to be credible messengers and who have the ability to tap into the information available in the community about conflicts that are about to erupt. What that means, he said, is that programs are hiring people with challenges of their own, and as a result, the trauma-informed approach that James described should also be used when hiring, supervising, and supporting the workers as much as the participants.

Butts also commented that the challenge he and his colleagues are facing when trying to evaluate programs such as Cure Violence and get a picture of what different programs emphasize is that just because they all have the same branding does not mean they are all doing the same thing. "There are variations among sites that happen because of the personalities of the people running the program or the number of people hired and their background," said Butts. He claimed there is "an epidemic of confirmation bias among these programs," and admitted he has his own biases about what makes these programs strong. What is needed, said Butts, is the time and resources to invest in enough research and fidelity measures to know which exact components and behaviors of the programs lead to the best outcomes. "We are far from understanding the huge assortment of variables that go into that mix," said Butts.

Antonia Clemente with the Healing Center, a domestic violence and gender justice organization, commented that none of the presentations mentioned violence against women and children and asked why that had not been part of the workshop's conversation. She also asked if Cure Violence and these other programs address the connections between gun violence and domestic violence. Webster acknowledged the importance of the issues Clemente raised and said that the Cure Violence Health Model was created to address gang violence more than other types of violence. That being said, he noted that Cure Violence clearly recognizes that partner violence is part of the social norms that accept violence in these communities and therefore is part of what the program tries to address. Domestic violence is just not the primary focus of this particular program. He noted that many of the concepts being discussed at this workshop are related to women's safety and intimate partner violence. Betty Lee Davis, a clinical social worker, added that other workshops have addressed partner violence.

Charles Branas of the University of Pennsylvania commented that while Cure Violence has spread to many cities around the country, he wondered how in the future it would be possible to pair this type of program with a university or scientific evaluation team early in the process. Butts replied that RWJF did that when it attached his evaluation team to the program early in its development. He added that RWJF has expressed an interest in knitting together evaluation and programmatic partners to have a common conversation. Webster added that the CDC's youth violence support center is the other major funder of research in this area.

Butts said the hospital component can be an incredibly powerful part of a violence intervention program if done well, but the political and economic power of the health sector can easily overwhelm the neighborhood base of what a Cure Violence program is supposed to be. "You do not want to professionalize it too much, but somehow there has to be a linking mechanism that allows the neighborhood-oriented credible messengers to feel comfortable interacting with the health industry," Butts explained. The best example of this that he has seen is in New Orleans, Louisiana, where there is an effective, respectful collaboration among law enforcement, the hospital, and residents in the neighborhood. The most important piece is that the police understand they should not interfere with or dilute the power of the neighborhood component, which requires cooperation and communication with the leadership of the police department. In contrast, he has heard stories in which the police try to undermine programs by walking up to workers onsite after a shooting, which destroys the trust the community has in these workers.

George Isham of HealthPartners wondered in relation to scaling and consistency if there is a need to bring in collaborators from business schools who could share what they know about creating consistent leadership and scaling interventions so that they are more reproducible across geographies and organizations. Webster thought that was an important point and said he is co-chair of a recently formed Safe Streets Baltimore advisory committee that includes people with just that expertise to help them think about program management. He noted the importance of working collaboratively with other experts to think about how to scale effective initiatives to address violence on a national scale.

An unidentified workshop participant asked the panelists to comment on the difficulty of paying the on-the-ground workers a salary commensurate with the difficulty and danger associated with their jobs in the community. Both Webster and Butts agreed this is a significant problem and both expressed dismay that these workers not only have a hard time getting paid what they deserve, but because these programs are often funded through city contracts, there can be gaps and delays in paying salaries. They also agreed this is an issue that will have to be addressed if these programs are to be sustainable, particularly given that the most effective workers, the ones who play a major role in the success of these programs, do not treat these as 9-to-5 professions. "We have to recognize just how challenging it is to do [these jobs] and support the workers. They are saving lives and we need to value them," said Webster.

Dorothy Indyk, a retired preventive medicine specialist, remarked that she is disappointed and distressed that the lessons learned over 30 years in the HIV field about the importance of integrating prevention and treatment are being relearned by this field. "No matter which conference I go to, I find the same problem. We are creating new siloes," said Indyk. She noted that while CDC has expanded its programs dramatically, it is still silo-based in terms of how it defines prevention. "We have to define prevention holistically across the life cycle. We are still doing acute-level interventions," she added.

An unidentified workshop participant asked if any of the evaluations of these programs have been able to identify how structural differences among different communities affect the ability of these interventions to be successful. Webster responded that research has so far made some general observations. It should be no surprise that if you are going to the places where the problem of gun violence is the worst, that these organizations will be the most stressed, have the least resources, and so on, said Webster. Another variable appears to be how overtaxed the organizations running these programs are and how truly committed they are to the community. He said he has seen the highest resourced organizations not do well when the commitment piece is missing.

Butts remarked that knowledge development in this area is restricted or impeded by the issue of data outcomes. He recounted a conversation he had with a physician who said he could say exactly how many cases of hepatitis B there were in his community from year to year. Butts replied to this physician that he does not have a state legislature deciding what hepatitis B is, nor is hepatitis B a different disease in every state. The definitions of violent crimes, the reporting rates, and the way that violent crimes are addressed differ across jurisdictions and communities. "It is very hard to know who has been violent or who will be violent, and that squishiness makes it hard to implement solid programs and evaluate them," said Butts.

6

Public Health and Law Enforcement Collaborations

The workshop's final panel session featured three presentations focused on how police departments are tackling the problem of community violence by collaborating with public health professionals and incorporating public health models and practices into policing. Steve Marans, the Harris Professor and director of the National Center for Children Exposed to Violence/Childhood Violent Trauma Center at the Yale Child Study Center, and director of the trauma service and professor of psychiatry at Yale School of Medicine, spoke about efforts to translate clinical observations about childhood violent trauma into effective interventions. John Markovic, senior social science analyst in the Office of Community Oriented Policing Services (COPS) at the U.S. Justice Department (DOJ), presented an overview of programs supported by his office. Medina Henry, associate director of training and technical assistance at the Center for Court Innovation, then described a collaborative initiative between the U.S. Department of Health and Human Services' Office of Minority Health and COPS aimed at preventing youth violence. An open discussion, moderated by Ted Corbin, associate professor in the department of emergency medicine at Drexel University School of Medicine, followed the three presentations. Highlights and main points made by individual speakers are in Box 6-1.

BOX 6-1
Highlights and Main Points Made by Individual Speakers[a]

- One lesson learned about trauma is that it is perhaps the most significant public health crisis the United States faces (Marans).
- Trauma often goes unrecognized, in children in particular, and when left untreated, the aftereffects of trauma can lead to well-established adverse consequences (Marans).
- The United States has the intellectual and financial resources to help children overcome the adverse effects of trauma and meet their full potential (Marans).
- A public health approach to violence reduction can be integrated with policing practices. Among the several existing frameworks that consider violence as a public health issue, a common thread is to focus on those who are most likely to be affected by violence and promote action as something that will benefit the common good, rather than as a strict law enforcement action (Markovic).
- Opportunities for youth development and leadership are a key aspect of the Minority Youth Violence Prevention intervention projects. Young people need to be given an opportunity to develop their own agency, and that is what each of the nine demonstration sites do very well (Henry).
- The grantees and the populations the Minority Youth Violence Prevention Initiative serve are diverse, as are the approaches and types of violence the initiatives are addressing. Some of the interventions target antisocial behaviors such as bullying, gang activities, violent crimes, homicides, and trauma. All of the sites focus on prosocial behavior, whether that is through police athletic league mentoring, healthy living, or other recreational activities (Henry).

[a] This list is the rapporteurs' summary of the main points made by individual speakers (noted in parentheses), and the statements have not been endorsed or verified by the National Academies of Sciences, Engineering, and Medicine.

TRANSLATING CLINICAL OBSERVATIONS INTO INTERVENTIONS FOR CHILDHOOD TRAUMA[1]

Steve Marans opened his presentation by saying that too often, human beings want quick fixes to disturbing problems. As a nation of creativity and innovations, there is often a desire to move quickly to scale interven-

[1] This section is the rapporteurs' synopsis of the presentation made by Steve Marans, the Harris Professor and director of the National Center for Children Exposed to Violence/Childhood Violent Trauma Center at the Yale Child Study Center, and director of the trauma service and professor of psychiatry at the Yale School of Medicine, and the statements have not been endorsed or verified by the National Academies of Sciences, Engineering, and Medicine.

tions without taking advantage of what has been learned along the way. An example, said Marans, is a failure to focus on trauma prevention.

The characteristics of trauma, he explained, are that it occurs when there is an overwhelming, unanticipated danger and feeling of helplessness that leaves an individual believing there is nothing to do to change, alter, or get away from the unanticipated event. In addition, there is an immobilization of the usual methods of defending oneself—the fight-or-flight response—and in fact, what usually happens in the acute moments of trauma is that an individual freezes. "We know that these experiences are undergirded and occur because of neurophysiologic dysregulation that compromises the way we are able to think, feel, and act," said Marans. "It is an important consideration to remember that when we are talking about a traumatic experience, we are actually talking about the ways our brains are able to function. That has an enormous impact on how we feel and what we do in response."

A clinical roadmap of trauma, said Marans, shows it occurs in phases: an acute phase lasting a few hours to a few days; the peritraumatic period lasting up to 3 months after the index event; and the chronic phase, characterized by the symptoms of PTSD and related disorders. Trauma can also have a delayed onset. The general symptoms of trauma are reexperiencing the index event, avoidance, and hyperarousal.

One lesson learned about trauma, said Marans, is that it is perhaps the most significant public health crisis the United States faces. This lesson, he said, is stressed in a report from the Attorney General's Task Force for Children Exposed to Violence (Listenbee et al., 2012) and by many other organizations that have studied psychological trauma related to violence. In children in particular, trauma often goes unrecognized, and when left untreated, the aftereffects of trauma can lead to well-established adverse consequences. Marans emphasized this last statement because it ties back to his opening remarks about failing to follow through on lessons learned. "We fail too often to go far enough upstream," said Marans. "We respond to the end-state result, which galvanizes and attracts our attention, but too often we are not going far enough upstream to think about prevention." By prevention, he added, he was referring to treatments that can enable someone to recover from trauma and not suffer horrible outcomes that can include perpetuating violence.

The number of children who experience multiple types of potentially traumatic impacts and experiences is enormous, said Marans. The numbers are so large, he believes, that it leads the public to feel there is nothing that can be done to stop trauma from affecting children. The consequence of putting blinders on with regard to this problem is that it exacerbates one of the strongest risk factors for experiencing poor outcomes after trauma—the failure of caregivers or the broader community to recognize the impact of trauma and provide social and familial support to the children who experience trauma.

The challenge to going upstream, as Marans put it, is to identify the children and families most impacted by potentially traumatic events. "How are non-mental health professionals, who actually respond to these situations, whether on the streets or in hospitals, schools, jails, or the criminal justice system, going to respond if they are not equipped [to identify trauma] and don't have the right partners [to address trauma]?" asked Marans. He noted that research on trauma has led to the development of standardized tools for identifying the symptoms of trauma, training methods to teach non-mental health professionals how to use these tools correctly, and clinical strategies for getting the right treatments to those in need. The issue, said Marans, is how to take these to scale.

In 1991, Marans and his fellow clinicians at the Yale Child Study Center, who he said were steeped in the development of human behavior and the impact of trauma, realized that the majority of children and families affected by trauma were never going to come in for treatment. "We were never going to meet them, and often when we would, it would be so far down the road that the damage had been done," said Marans. In response to this recognition, Marans and his colleagues reached out to the New Haven, Connecticut, police department, which he said was also frustrated with the 911-driven, post-incident response to violence that was not making a dent in the problem. The result was a collaboration that involved taking advantage of police authority and using it benignly to step in to help people, precisely at the time when they are not functioning optimally, and start them down the road to recovery.

Today, all police officers in New Haven and the other communities where this program has been implemented are trained on the intersection of child development, human functioning, trauma, and community policing, and participating clinicians are trained in the basics of policing. Similar to the police, clinicians are on call 24 hours per day and respond with police when notified there has been some potentially traumatic event. For the past 25 years, Marans and his clinical colleagues have been meeting weekly with the New Haven police to discuss the cases they have worked on together as a means of examining the wide range of intervention strategies needed to ensure optimal recovery.

In addition to the on-call service, the program has repeated follow-up visits with those potentially affected by trauma. "We identify different roles that different players—not just the police, but social services, medical providers, the schools, and others—can play in helping kids and families get back on their feet," said Marans. Together, the police and clinicians also canvass neighborhoods after an event that has impacted an entire neighborhood to let the community know their problem is not being ignored and to provide information about what the communities can do to help one another and their children and to connect them with available resources.

When Marans and his colleagues did a study of the impact of this type of intervention on women who had been victims of domestic violence in front of their children, they found that women who were part of the outreach group, as opposed to women who were getting the standard 911-driven police response, called police more often to address later incidents of violence. Moreover, these calls were not 911 calls, but regular calls to the neighborhood police whom they had come to know through regular contacts in the community. In addition, the number of children who were directed to trauma-related services was nearly two-thirds higher in the outreach group compared to the standard response group. A consumer satisfaction survey showed that the biggest reason for the dramatic increase in calls and use of services was that these women believed the police were ready and willing to support them. Marans noted that one lesson he and his colleagues have learned from their work in New Haven and in response to the September 11, 2001, terrorist attacks, Hurricane Katrina, and the Newtown school shootings, is that one group of professionals or one set of community members cannot tackle the enormous challenges that arise when individuals and entire communities are overwhelmed by trauma.

Marans and his colleagues have recently developed a toolkit and 2-day training in collaboration with the International Association of Chiefs of Police and DOJ. They are now hoping to get funding to make the toolkit and training available to law enforcement agencies nationwide. The goal, he said, is to train police officers who respond to these horrific and potentially traumatic situations with something to offer the affected individuals that can benefit their lives. Too often, police responding to tragedies believe there is nothing they can do to help the innocent victims of these highly traumatic events. "I think our experience as a country is not dissimilar," said Marans. "We look away when we talk about trauma because we are not informed that we are not helpless to respond to what we do have control over." The United States, he added, has the intellectual and financial resources to help children overcome the adverse effects of trauma and meet their full potential.

Marans and his colleagues have also developed an early intervention aimed at preventing the long-term disorders that can develop in children when trauma is left untreated (Marans, 2013; Marans et al., 2012). The intervention lasts from five to eight sessions and is based on a family-strengthening model. It is meant to be delivered to children from ages 3 to 8 during the peritraumatic period or after the recent disclosure of sexual or physical abuse. Marans said the intervention reduces posttraumatic reactions, helps the children regain control of their emotions, increases communication between children and their caregivers, and leads to an effective decrease in the development of PTSD of 65 percent in comparison to standard of care. In addition, those receiving the intervention are 73 percent less likely to develop a broader range of posttraumatic reactions as compared to standard approaches.

OFFICE OF COMMUNITY ORIENTED POLICING SERVICES[2]

COPS was established in 1994 as part of the Crime Control and Law Enforcement Act of 1994 with a mission of advancing public safety through community policing, said John Markovic. Community policing, he explained, focuses on collaborative efforts to prevent and respond to crime, social disorder, and fear or crime, and it gets away from the idea of policing as strict law enforcement. The community policing era, he added, started around 1984 when a group of progressive police chiefs and academics came up with the idea that the police needed to reconnect with their communities. The preceding era, known as the legalistic era, was characterized by a strict adherence to rules, procedures, and regulations that developed as a reasonable response to police corruption scandals. Community policing, said Markovic, has always existed in some form, though its emphasis and priorities have changed over the years.

One of the mainstays of the COPS program is its hiring grant program for law enforcement agencies. Since 1994, COPS has provided some $14 billion in funding to enable more than 13,000 law enforcement agencies to put some 126,000 community policing officers on city streets, procure technology, and develop demonstration projects and tools, Markovic explained. Approximately 76 percent of the nation's law enforcement agencies have received COPS grant funds. Except for 2009, when stimulus funds were allocated for hiring more police officers, COPS hiring grants per year have averaged between $200 million and $400 million. COPS also has a community policing development program and a grant program to promote demonstration projects, training, and research on advancing community policing. More recently, COPS has provided funding to state police agencies to support task forces to deal specifically with methamphetamine and heroin use. COPS also supports a DOJ-wide Tribal Technical Assistance Program to make it easier for tribal police departments to apply for and receive funding from DOJ.

[2] This section is the rapporteurs' synopsis of the presentation made John Markovic, senior social science analyst in the Office of Community-Oriented Policing Services at the U.S. Department of Justice, and the statements have not been endorsed or verified by the National Academies of Sciences, Engineering, and Medicine.

In December 2014, President Obama signed an Executive Order establishing the President's Task Force on 21st Century Policing with the mission of promoting effective crime reduction while building public trust. Composed of a diverse group of experts, including activists, police chiefs, academics, civil rights organizations, and union officials, the task force developed a set of six pillars around which it organized its recommendations:

1. Building Trust and Legitimacy
2. Policy and Oversight
3. Technology and Social Media
4. Community Policing and Crime Reduction
5. Training and Education
6. Officer Safety and Wellness

The task force's recommendations focused on strategies to reduce crime in a manner that did not alienate the community, and in fact, would enrich the community and minimize the collateral damage that sometimes results from strict law enforcement actions. The recommendations also emphasized making improvements in the training and education of police officers and focusing on officer safety and wellness given that policing is a stressful profession.

One recommendation, for example, called for law enforcement agencies to "collaborate with community members to develop policies and strategies in communities and neighborhoods disproportionately affected by crime for deploying resources that aim to reduce crime by improving relationships, greater community engagement, and cooperation" (President's Task Force on 21st Century Policing, 2015). Other recommendations, said Markovic, also emphasized collaboration and community building, procedural justice, and the use of a guardianship model of policing rather than a warrior model. Markovic noted that since the early days of COPS, its hiring programs emphasized recruiting and hiring police officers motivated by a spirit of service rather than a call to "action."

A public health approach to violence reduction can be integrated with policing practices, said Markovic. He noted that among the several existing frameworks that consider violence as a public health issue, a common thread is to focus on those who are most likely to be affected by violence and promote action as something that will benefit the common good, rather than as a strict law enforcement action. A strict law enforcement model, he said, "to put it very bluntly or crudely in the interest of time, it is finding out who the bad guys are, knowing who the good guys are, and putting the bad guys away." Markovic went on to say that is not the model that reflects modern-day policing and it is not the model that they promote. Both the World Health Organization and CDC stress the necessity of relying on data-driven approaches to address community violence that follow the public health model of identifying and prioritizing problems, identifying the risk and protective factors, developing and testing prevention strategies, and ensuring widespread adoption with continued evaluation of effectiveness. Markovic noted that an important aspect of community policing is that it does not just focus on the offender, but also on the environment in which violence occurs and the people who experience it.

Several of the tools used by police to identify risk are hot-spot policing and social network analysis. Markovic noted that maps of violence hot spots and comorbidities such as low education levels, a shortage of services, obesity, and cardiovascular disease usually overlap in distressed communities down to the block level. Social network analysis is used as an advanced analytics tool to enable a focused deterrence approach to addressing community violence.

Social network analysis relies on the observation that violence follows a disease contagion model, in which individuals who are associated with people who are the causes or victims of violence are much more likely to become victims of violence themselves or to be shooters, said Markovic. The focused deterrence approach means that the individuals identified as potentially most responsible for violence are approached by the police and warned of the legal consequences if they do not stop. Officers also contact other stakeholders—family members, clergy, prosecutors, and others—and bring them together to provide support.

Another strategy called the Cardiff Model for Violence Prevention, Markovic explained, relies on partnerships and public health to show that integrating emergency department and police data can help locate violence hot spots. Developed in Wales, originators of the Cardiff model identified hot spots of violence, which become focus areas in which to apply prevention strategies and produce significant reductions in violence (Florence et al., 2011). The Cardiff model identified neighborhoods surrounding drinking spots as the most common hot spots for violence. The solution was to have the drinking establishments replace their glassware with cups because incidents in Cardiff tend to involve stabbings rather than shootings. The police also went through the hot-spot neighborhoods and removed debris that could be used as weapons. An assessment of this approach showed that it did reduce violence compared to other areas in which standard policing was in effect.

Another approach is risk terrain modeling (Caplan and Kennedy, 2016), which is being offered free to analysts and police agencies, said Markovic. Public health officials have used risk terrain modeling to find areas with an elevated incidence of child abuse and neglect. This type of predictive modeling identifies crime generators and crime inhibitors in the environment to forecast where crime is more likely to occur in the future.

The "Fit Zone" project in East Palo Alto, California, said Markovic, is another example of a public health approach that successfully reduced crime (Lawrence et al., 2012; Markovic, 2012). There, the police department identified areas where there were high volumes of gunshots by using traditional police data and shot-spotter data. The police helped organize community physical activities such as walking, biking, and even Zumba workouts to take back the neighborhood and create an environment that felt safe. An evaluation of the program found it reduced crime significantly in some neighborhoods.

MINORITY YOUTH VIOLENCE PREVENTION INITIATIVES[3]

In 2014, DOJ and the U.S. Department of Health and Human Services' Office of Minority Health issued an innovative joint solicitation that is now funding nine demonstration sites that promote a public health and community policing approach to violence prevention with minority youths. Medina Henry, an associate director for training and technical assistance at the Center for Court Innovation, described the 3-year Minority Youth Violence Prevention Initiative.

Howard explained that the official goals of the project are to

- reduce violent crimes against minority youth;
- reduce community violence and crimes perpetrated by minority youth;
- improve academic outcomes for participants;
- reduce negative encounters with law enforcement;
- increase access to public health and/or social services; and
- improve coordination, collaboration, and linkages among agencies.

In their proposals, applicants for the grants were required to include public health and law enforcement partners. They also had to identify where violence was occurring in their communities, list the strategies that had been used in the past to address violence in those areas, and detail what interventions they were proposing to reduce violence among the young people in their communities. The nine grantees selected for

[3] This section is the rapporteurs' synopsis of the presentation made by Medina Henry, associate director of training and technical assistance at the Center for Court Innovation, and the statements have not been endorsed or verified by the National Academies of Sciences, Engineering, and Medicine.

the Minority Youth Prevention Initiative[4] include two community-based organizations, two health-related organizations, a hospital, a health department, a police department, a district attorney's office, and a city/county. The sites are in different areas of the country and include diverse populations. Two of the sites are where large populations of refugees have resettled, which Henry explained affects the type of violence that people in those communities have experienced and the interventions aimed at those particular communities.

Henry's role in the project is to serve as a technical assistance provider to support the grantees. She helps them to identify staffing and training resources, advises them on the evidence-based practices being implemented, and how to identify risks within their programming. Henry said she spent a great deal of time encouraging the sites to be intentional about their work and the populations they are serving. She has also helped the sites identify proxies for various outcomes, such as negative encounters with police, and to work with the sites to improve coordination, collaboration, and linkages among agencies, which Henry said is challenging, but also likely to be the most sustainable element of the project.

The grantees and the populations they serve are diverse, said Henry, as are the approaches and types of violence the initiatives address. Some interventions target antisocial behaviors such as bullying, gang activities, violent crimes, homicides, and trauma. All sites focus on prosocial behavior, whether through police athletic league mentoring, healthy living, or other recreational activities. The intervention sites include hospital-based, school-based, and community-based programming. Some of the school-based projects focus on bullying, she noted, and several of the hospital-based programs collaborate with community policing efforts. At least one site deals with the trauma in families who have had a family member killed by violence. Henry noted that while dealing with trauma is not an explicit goal for these grants, it is impossible to talk about violence without addressing trauma, too. In some sites, she said, a trauma-informed approach to intervention, implementation, and development is an explicit component of the program (e.g., Children in Trauma Intervention, Cincinnati, Ohio; and Youth ALIVE!, Oakland, California), while others do not explicitly mention trauma but it is part of their work.[5]

In Minneapolis, where a sizable community resettled from Southeast Asia, Asian Media Access organized Shop-with-a-Cop, said Henry, as a

[4] For more information about the initiatives, see http://www.courtinnovation.org/minority-youth-violence-prevention-initiative (accessed August 22, 2016).

[5] For more information on specific sites, as well as links to podcasts, see http://www.courtinnovation.org/minority-youth-violence-prevention-initiative (accessed November 2, 2016).

way to engage the community so that youth and police officers get to know each other on a more intimate level as police officers support these youth in getting education supplies. Through a parallel series of workshops, Asian Media Access provides training to law enforcement about cultural awareness and does community education to different immigrant groups around civic engagement and the role of law enforcement. Toward the end of the workshop series, Asian Media Access brings the police and the community together for an open dialogue at which community members can ask questions and law enforcement can explain policies and procedures. Henry noted that there is a general lack of understanding in these communities of what the police do and are required to do, so this is a way for both communities to learn more about each other.

At some of the sites, such as in Cincinnati, law enforcement officers serve as the facilitators, leading workshops and physical recreational activities and acting as formal or informal mentors. In Cincinnati, a youth organization provides police officers, who largely come from the youth services unit, with training on mentorship. Often, Henry explained, the role of law enforcement is not primarily to support young people, so the police learn how to engage with youth. "I think we take it for granted that people know how to talk to a young person and that just is not necessarily the case," said Henry.

Programs may also focus on youth basketball leagues or community service. In the beginning, some programs that include developing supportive relationships between police officers and youth can be difficult, and sometimes a neutral third party facilitator needs to be involved to model appropriate interactions between the police officer and students. However, over the course of a semester, the officers and students get to know each other and build trust. Building on those relationships, there can be larger outreach and community engagement efforts through which youth bring their family and friends to engage with law enforcement differently and build trust and communication in the community.

With regard to the trauma-informed initiatives, the Cincinnati Police Children in Trauma Intervention program includes structured military drills for physical fitness (it is not a boot camp). There is a trauma specialist on site and all of the officers that participate get trauma training. Youth ALIVE! in Oakland, California, developed the Screening Tool for Awareness and Relief of Trauma.[6] The screening tool was developed to address the needs of young men of color who disproportionately experience trauma, yet current approaches and responses to their particular needs are limited, said Henry. Youth ALIVE! has a trauma specialist on

---

[6] For more information, see http://www.youthalive.org/wp-content/uploads/2016/06/Trauma-Project-Clinical-Two-Pager-June-2015.pdf (accessed November 2, 2016).

site and also facilitates trainings for their staff, partners and others in the community. In Sacramento, California, the Health Education Council participates in a statewide initiative to inform all of their systems about trauma-informed care, education, the justice system, and other systems that impact the lives of youth.

Henry concluded her talk with common trends and promising practices she has identified over the first 18 months of this program. Multisector collaborations are nothing new, but many of the grantees have a convener, a designated person who brings collaborators to the table, organizes ways of thinking, and helps develop the shared vision, goals, and action plans. These are working groups, said Henry, and at most of the sites the collaborators have been working with one another for a long time, creating a certain level of trust and the ability to get key decision makers to the table quickly.

Opportunities for youth development and leadership are a key aspect of these interventions, said Henry. "You have to give a young person an opportunity to develop their own agency, and I think many of the sites do that very well," she said. Another programmatic practice that she has seen at many sites is an intentional process for engaging the guardians or family members of the young people enrolled in these programs. "It is probably one of the hardest things and one of the challenges that many of the sites face in terms of consistently and actively engaging and getting a response from guardians and families," said Henry. Often these adults are overwhelmed by the many responsibilities they have in their lives. These efforts to do outreach do lead to positive results, she added.

The final promising practice Henry has seen among the grantees is the development of strategic intervention based on shared data and information. Sharing data may be hard, she said, but the grantees are addressing that challenge and their interventions are the better for it. She also noted that just having conversations about sharing information has led to some ideas about other interventions to try. She noted in closing that the program's website (http://www.courtinnovation.org/minority-youth-violence-prevention-initiative [accessed January 5, 2017]) has links to the nine grantees as well as podcasts that feature the different grantees and their partners and additional information about the tools and strategies the grantees are using in their communities.

DISCUSSION

Ted Corbin started the discussion by asking how such amazing examples of collaborations at the local level between health care and public safety and at the federal level between health and justice come to be. Marans replied, "Being in pain and having humility," and Markovic said it was partly by planning and partly by necessity to fill gaps. A big part of creating these collaborations, said Markovic, is people who are open to learning from different disciplines and understanding how approaches can be complementary instead of siloed.

Betty Lee Davis first commented that she sees this workshop's focus on trauma as an important first step in stopping the transmission of violence. She then asked the panelists to comment on the role of racism in explaining why resources are not widely available to implement these interventions in communities of color given the long-standing attention given to youth violence as a public health problem. Marans replied that the unfolding history and legacy of discrimination in this country is one in which a disproportionately high level of certain kinds of illnesses and traumas are prevalent in communities of color.

Markovic replied by describing a study in which police officers were shown pictures of men holding guns or cellphones and asked if they would shoot or not. "As might be expected, the respondents are quicker to mistakenly identify cellphones as guns when the subjects are African American or other minorities." This is a manifestation, he explained, of implicit bias, which also exists with regard to characteristics such as sexual orientation, political orientations, and obesity. The interesting thing about this study, however, was that the results held true across all groups, including among African American officers and students. He then noted there is evidence emerging to show that once an individual recognizes implicit bias, there are ways of changing behavior for the better.

Davis also asked the panelists if secondary trauma and the effects of law enforcement's exposure to violence is contributing to the police-involved incidents that are now getting so much attention. Markovic responded that he believes that there is recognition that law enforcement officers are experiencing long-term effects of the stress. He and his colleagues have been working with law enforcement on what is known as procedural justice, the recognition that people obey the law because they find it procedurally just and generally fair, and not merely because they fear the consequences. There are two elements of procedural justice in this training. One is outward facing—that police officers and police administration should be fair to citizens in their interactions—and this concept is now being applied to new training procedures that are attempting to change the use of force and that stress the sanctity of life for all people, including the officers themselves. He also noted that in the early 2000s, the New York Police Department had a courtesy, professionalism, and respect training program. Customer satisfaction surveys showed that even when people received traffic tickets or citations for other violations, they reported feeling they had been treated fairly by the police. However, there were differences in how people felt by race and age, but they were not as pronounced as the differences found when a random sampling of people is asked for their general opinions of the police.

The other element of training is internal procedural justice, which addresses how officers may find it hard to be fair with the public when they are constantly in a job where they believe they have been treated unfairly. Markovic said that officer safety and wellness was one of the pillars presented in the President's Task Force on 21st Century Policing (2014) report. There is a need, he said, to be proactive and develop physical and mental health programs for officers to help them deal with the stress of being on the streets, particularly for those who patrol high-crime neighborhoods.

At the same time, Markovic added, programs are needed to help police officers recognize the symptoms of their own stress so they seek help. As an example, he described a Milwaukee Police Department program funded by COPS in which officers were trained to monitor their heart rates as an indicator of stress and use several techniques to reduce stress. There is evidence from the U.S. military, he said, showing that such methods not only reduce stress, but also reduce risk factors for cardiovascular disease and PTSD and improve sleep and general well-being.

Marans took a different perspective on this issue, though he agreed that more attention needs to be paid to self-care in all stressful professions and particularly those professions in which a person's life is on the line. That said, he noted there are many high-stress professions with high rates of addiction and alcoholism, but it is unknown to what extent the failure to recover from trauma plays a role in that relationship. He also said that he has been to thousands of bloody murder scenes and as far as he is aware, he has never experienced the symptoms of PTSD and believes the reason is training and support. Police officers receive training and support to deal with murders, and this is completely different from the average citizen who is unprepared for a traumatic event, said Marans.

Another difference between police officers and the public that many in the civilian population do not appreciate is that the police do not go on service calls to celebrate the joys of life and the successes of love. Instead, they experience a steady diet, day in and day out, of confrontations and failures of life that can lead to the feeling that they are ineffective. "If we equip police officers to be able to be effective and feel effective, it is stunning the extent to which the blinders come off and the roles of being effective agents and supporting people getting back on their feet, and protecting lives is mobilized," said Marans.

Pamela Russo commented that RWJF is beginning to invest heavily in what it calls trauma-informed care for children and for high-using patients who are homeless or have a substance abuse disorder or mental illness. She noted, too, that there are trauma-informed schools and even a community in Georgia that refers to itself as a trauma-informed community. Her question for Marans was whether he thinks that trauma-informed interventions will work at a later point in life, that is, long after the traumatic event or events occurred. She also asked, with regard to children, if the same treatment can be used again if a child experiences a subsequent traumatic event. Marans replied that the key to treating trauma is to remember that every individual is different in the way they experience and react to traumatic events. He noted there have been studies done with young boys who display violent behavior that have found that these boys are overstimulated by trauma. The analogy he used was of a football team of 12-year-olds playing as a National Football League team. "There is an imbalance, and over time, that imbalance results in compromised functioning and capacity that can lead to serious illness," said Marans. What is important, he concluded, is to demonstrate equity and justice by treating each child and each adult as an individual and find out what specific treatments will fit that individual's needs.

With regard to whether it is possible to treat the effects of trauma long after the traumatic event, Marans replied that there are well-established treatments for adults that can relieve and decrease PTSD even after it is well established. He noted that PTSD is not the only outcome of trauma—poor frustration tolerance and an inability to concentrate in school are two other conditions resulting from the lack of support and compensation for the damage done by trauma.

An unidentified workshop participant remarked that the programs Henry described seem to be working hard to build solidarity and break down the "us versus them" mentality between young people and police officers. She then asked Henry if the programs are also working to connect these young people to employment or training opportunities, and Henry replied that every one of the nine sites has a component that connects young people to educational support and internships. Some sites, she said, are developing their own in-house programs, and others are working with outside organizations. The West Palm Beach site's Village Initiative, for example, works with the city, business development partners, and their vocational and educational partners to create job fairs. The message this program is sending is that they want local businesses to invest in the young people in the community and that they will work to train them so that they can become good employees. Consistent across all of the nine sites, said Henry, is consideration of the broader conditions these communities are facing with regard to access to quality food, good housing, employment, and education.

7

Reflections on the Day

The traditional conclusion to this roundtable's workshops is for the roundtable members, as well as other workshop participants, to offer their reflections and reactions to the day. "It is very difficult to do work in this area and do it well, but it is really important to do it." said Thomas LaVeist of The George Washington University. "I was struck by how diligent the researchers are in trying to bring rigor to what is an extremely difficult topic to study well." He also noted that violence can be a violence prevention strategy in that reacting quickly to an ambiguous threat can be lifesaving because the one time that response is wrong, an encounter could be fatal. In some ways, he said, violence is often seen as being pathological or indicative of a mental health condition, but in fact it could illustrate a healthy brain's response to an unhealthy context.

LaVeist commented that moving people out of their neighborhoods to move them into opportunity does not sound like a successful policy because inevitably there will be individuals who are not moved and as a result have even less opportunity. He also said it is unfortunate to think of the problem of violence in terms of hot spots and hot people because in his view they are two sides of the same coin. "We need to have strategies that focus on place and we need to have strategies that focus on people," said LaVeist.

LaVeist's final comments were in response to an earlier comment about the workshop not addressing domestic violence. He said the workshop planning committee decided to contextualize this workshop in a particular way by focusing on everyday structural violence that has disproportionate impacts on communities of color living in poverty. He also remarked that male-on-male violence was a narrative thread that came through in the workshop, but there are other gendered perspectives that this workshop did not address that could be a topic for a future workshop.

Mary Pittman of the Public Health Institute remarked that John Rich's theoretical framework on racism and violence was a good introduction to the workshop. She then noted that the interventions described at the workshop are long-term solutions that need sustainable funding. That funding needs to support better pay for those individuals who are taking on these dangerous roles as violence interrupters. She also commented that there were so many sectors and interventions discussed that a mapping exercise might help prioritize where to apply specific interventions. Other points she raised were the importance of having trusted players in the community and the link between trauma and violence. She also said she was somewhat surprised that the faith community was not mentioned much in the discussions and that she found the final panel framing of the relationship between the justice system and violence as a welcome approach.

Marthe Gold of The New York Academy of Medicine commented that the presentations emphasized the link between the environment and violence, a connection that fits into the broader discussion about determinants of health, but the idea of hot people described by DeVone Boggan was a new concept to her. That idea got her to thinking about how hot people live everywhere, come in every color, and come from every culture and how many there might still be even if the nation could magically erase the deprivation these communities face. "What do we do with them? How do we reconcile the fact that there are people that you do not change, who are intractable, who for whatever reasons, will always be sour on the world?" she asked. She also wondered what those attending the workshop could do to help create pressure to diminish the role of guns in American society and to engage the media to become more attuned to the losses that everyone suffers—not just privileged communities—when violence occurs.

Lourdes Rodríguez of the New York State Health Foundation commented on the parallels between hot people and high users in the health care system and how thinking about hot people in that way might lead to new solutions. She also drew another parallel between the services available for veterans returning home from combat to help them deal with the effects of trauma and individuals returning to the community who have been incarcerated. She wondered if society could suspend its biases regarding the latter if the nation could then think about ways of helping those individuals heal the effects of the traumas they have experienced in life. Rodríguez's final comment regarded the idea of characterizing the young people arriving at emergency departments as not having had caring adults in their lives. It may be that the adults in their lives are working 80 hours a week at two jobs to try to support their families.

Phyllis Meadows of The Kresge Foundation and the University of Michigan said she felt a sense of failure and hope after the day's presentations. She also thought about the young people who were the focus of the day's conversations and how society has created an image of them that gives others permission to walk away from them. "What I heard today was clear justification for why we cannot walk away from this topic," said Meadows. Her sense of failure comes from not knowing how to move other people to pay attention to these young people and not knowing how to move from talking to action. An important realization for her was that these young people have their own stories and that the individuals most responsible for violence are victims as well. "There are so many narratives in this, from the person who commits the violent act to the person who experiences it, to the family," said Meadows. It is important for their voices to be heard and their stories to be told. Her final comment, speaking as someone who works for a foundation that provides support for programs, was to consider what changes need to be made to make violence reduction programs no longer necessary. She commented that foundations are thinking about how to take a systems approach to these problems, and hopes that in the future more attention focuses on policies and systems: medical, justice, and others that contribute to the violence in communities.

Samara Ford, an undergraduate student at Harvard College, remarked that as someone interested in public health, she was inspired to hear experts talking about the topic of community violence at a workshop. One of her takeaway messages was the need to look at the intersection of self-worth and violence given the likelihood that if a young person feels his or her life has potential, that person will not put his or her life at risk. Her final comment was to remember that the discussion about community violence as a population health issue should also include the LGBTQ community, which is often the object of violence and suffering the health consequences of experiencing that violence.

George Isham of HealthPartners commented on the peace quilt hanging behind the podium that was created by children of Lutheran Church of the Good Shepherd, where the workshop was held. One of the squares said "Peace Begins with Me," and he commented on the optimism contained in that statement. The statement also made him wonder if peace is the opposite of violence. He then noted that in the aftermath of the June 12 Orlando nightclub shooting, some of the resulting television and political commentary distorted that incident into a single issue or self-aggrandizing rationales. "The country could use the reminder that this is a complex issue," said Isham. "One of the opportunities we have is to draw attention to that fact and draw on the expertise that we have heard during the course of the day."

Steve Smith from the University of Florida and a National Academy of Medicine Anniversary Fellow commented on how easy it is to be pessimistic about violence in society and how scary the topic of violence is for young people in the United States. However, he was impressed with the optimism espoused at this workshop that comes from these successful programs. "I think it reinforces the idea that we have to encourage and help facilitate these home-grown, community-driven interventions," said Smith. He suggested there might be an opportunity to have a workshop at which programs demonstrating successful population health interventions were published as a guide to others wanting to start programs.

Bobby Milstein of ReThink Health commented on the idea that the consequences of discrimination and racism unfairly disadvantages some communities and advantages others, but they also sap the strength of the entire nation. In his opinion, there has not been enough research done to identify how the strength of the nation is diminished by racism and discrimination, and he would like to hear more about that. He noted that there is a great deal of money invested in the prison-industrial complex because of the way the nation criminalizes violence while at the same time there are these many programs desperate for funding that create real value. "People who otherwise would have died are now here, families are better connected, there is just enormous value surrounding the things that we heard today, but not necessarily connected to the larger value equation, as it were," said Milstein. His sense is that these promising initiatives are being conducted on a shoestring despite the massive size of the problem. "I think it would be marvelous to learn a little bit more about the scope of the problem and its economics relative to the resources that are going to make a difference," he said.

Milstein also remarked that nonviolence is a discipline that has to be taught and learned and that nonviolence has saved many lives in addressing injustice. He wondered, then, when the nation lost its connection to non-violence. In his opinion, nonviolence can reconnect thriving economies that are more inclusive. In that vein, he commended the *Boston Globe*, which in the wake of the Orlando shooting published a list of tools for stopping gun violence (*Boston Globe*, 2016). "This is a major newspaper taking a stand in a way that is not just reporting the problem, but saying it has got to stop and here is how. It is just a remarkable landmark that, to me, is a move away from just observing this dynamic and saying if it is going to stop it is going to have to be people taking a stand and saying this as they have never done before in a spirit of nonviolence," said Milstein. He also applauded Connecticut Senator Chris Murphy's (D-CT) filibuster in the Senate on June 15, 2016, to demand action on gun control. LaVeist thanked Milstein for mentioning the filibuster and thought it important to acknowledge what was happening in Congress.

Speaking as a member of the clergy, Gary Gunderson of the Wake Forest School of Medicine commented that there are some quarter of a million congregations in the United States, and probably 99 percent of them do not engage these issues even though they would be well organized to do so. Rather than assuming that unless there is government intervention, change will not happen, Gunderson said, "There is very powerful testimony here that if you can be relevant and tenacious and follow the way that every single faith tradition has ever spoken to, you can shift the pattern of these most profound and intractable problems."

To close the workshop, Sanne Magnan commented that during the workshop, "We have felt emotions of sadness and anger, and yet out of all of that has also come hope."

Appendix A

References

Boston Globe. 2016. Make it stop. *Boston Globe*. June 15. http://apps.bostonglobe.com/graphics/2016/06/make-it-stop (accessed September 6, 2016).

Branas, C. C. 2010. Injury prevention in the developing world. *Italian Journal of Public Health* 7(2):72-75.

Branas, C. C., R. A. Cheney, J. M. MacDonald, V. W. Tam, T. D. Jackson, and T. R. Ten Have. 2011. A difference-in-differences analysis of health, safety, and greening vacant urban space. *American Journal of Epidemiology*. doi: 10.1093/aje/kwr273.

Brayne, S. 2014. Surveillance and system avoidance: Criminal justice contact and institutional attachment. *American Sociological Review* 79(3):367-391.

Caplan, J. M., and L. W. Kennedy. 2016. *Risk terrain modeling: Crime prediction and risk reduction*. Berkeley: University of California Press.

Card, A. J. 2012. Sustainability of public health programs. *American Journal of Public Health* 102(5):776-777; author reply 777.

Corbin, T. J., J. Purtle, L. J. Rich, J. A. Rich, E. J. Adams, G. Yee, and S. L. Bloom. 2013. The prevalence of trauma and childhood adversity in an urban, hospital-based violence intervention program. *Journal of Health Care for the Poor and Underserved* 24(3):1021-1030.

Feldmeyer, B. 2010. The effects of racial/ethnic segregation on Latino and Black homicide. *Social Quarterly* 51(4):600-623.

Felitti, V. J., R.F. Anda, D. Nordenberg, D. F. Williamson, A. M. Spitz, V. Edwards, M. P. Koss, and J. S. Marks. 1998. Relationship of childhood abuse and household dysfunction to many of the leading causes of death in adults. The Adverse Childhood Experiences (ACE) study. *American Journal of Preventive Medicine* 14(4):245-258.

Florence, C., J. Shepherd, I. Brennan, and T. Simon. 2011. Effectiveness of anonymised information sharing and use in health service, police, and local government partnership for preventing violence related injury: Experimental study and time series analysis. *BMJ* 342:d3313.

Frieden, T. R. 2010. A framework for public health action: The health impact pyramid. *American Journal of Public Health* 100(4):590-595.

Garvin, E., C. C. Branas, S. Keddem, J. Sellman, and C. Cannuscio. 2012. More than just an eyesore: Local insights and solutions on vacant land and urban health. *Journal of Urban Health* 12(7):9782-9787.

Geller, A., J. Fagan, T. Tyler, and B. G. Link. 2014. Aggressive policing and the mental health of young urban men. *American Journal of Public Health* 104(12):2321-2327.

IOM (Institute of Medicine). 2014. *Supporting a movement for health and health equity: Lessons from social movements: Workshop summary*. Washington, DC: The National Academies Press. https://doi.org/10.17226/18751.

IOM. 2015. *The role and potential of communities in population health improvement: Workshop summary*. Washington, DC: The National Academies Press. https://doi.org/10.17226/18946.

IOM and NRC (National Research Council). 2013a. *Contagion of violence: Workshop summary*. Washington, DC: The National Academies Press. https://doi.org/10.17226/13489.

IOM and NRC. 2013b. *Priorities for research to reduce the threat of firearm-related violence*. Washington, DC: The National Academies Press. https://doi.org/10.17226/18319.

Jacoby, S. F., L. Tach, T. Guerra, D. J. Wiebe, and T. S. Richmond. 2016. The health status and well-being of low-resource, housing-unstable, single-parent families living in violent neighbourhoods in Philadelphia, Pennsylvania. *Health and Social Care in the Community*. doi: 10.1111/hsc.12345.

Jones, C. P. 2000. Levels of racism: A theoretic framework and a gardener's tale. *American Journal of Public Health* 90(8):1212-1215.

Jones, C. P. 2002. Confronting institutionalized racism. *Phylon (1960-)* 50(1/2):7-22.

Katz, B., and J. Bradley. 2013. *The metropolitan revolution: How cities and metros are fixing broken politics and fragile economy*. Washington, DC: Brookings Institution Press.

Keizer, K., S. Lindenberg, and L. Steg. 2008. The spreading of disorder. *Science* 322(5908):1681-1685.

Kondo, M. C., S. Han, B. C. Hohl, and C. C. Branas. 2015a. Effects of greening and community reuse of vacant lots on crime. *Urban Studies* 52(15):1-17.

Kondo, M. C., D. Keene, B. C. Hohl, J. M. MacDonald, and C. C. Branas. 2015b. A difference-in-differences study of the effects of a new abandoned building remediation strategy on safety. *PLOS ONE* 10(7):e0129582.

Lawrence, S., R. A. Davis, and B. Jacobson. 2012. Using public health strategies to reduce violence in "hot spots" in East Palo Alto, California. *Geography and Public Safety* 3(2):5-8.

Liebschutz, J., R. Saitz, V. Brower, T. M. Keane, C. Lloyd-Travaglini, T. Averbuch, and J. H. Samet. 2007. PTSD in urban primary care: High prevalence and low physician recognition. *Journal of General Internal Medicine* 22(6):719-726.

Listenbee, Jr., R. L., J. Torre, G. Boyle, S. W. Cooper, S. Deer, D. T. Durfee, T. James, A. Lieberman, R. Macy, S. Marans, J. McDonnell, G. Mendoza, and A. Taguba. 2012. *Report of the Attorney General's National Task Force on Children Exposed to Violence*. Washington, DC: U.S. Department of Justice.

Ludwig, J., L. Sanbonmatsu, L. Gennetian, E. Adam, G. J. Duncan, L. F. Katz, R. C. Kessler, J. R. Kling, S. T. Lindau, R. C. Whitaker, and T. W. McDade. 2011. Neighborhoods, obesity, and diabetes—a randomized social experiment. *New England Journal of Medicine* 365(16):1509-1519.

Ludwig, J., G. J. Duncan, L. A. Gennetian, L. F. Katz, R. C. Kessler, J. R. Kling, and L. Sanbonmatsu. 2012. Neighborhood effects on the long-term well-being of low-income adults. *Science* 337(6101):1505-1510.

Marans, S. 2013. Phenomena of childhood trauma and expanding approaches to early intervention. *International Journal of Applied Psychoanalytic Studies* 10(3):247-266.

Marans, S., D. Smolover, and H. Hahn. 2012. Responding to child trauma: Theory, programs, and policy. In *Handbook of juvenile forensic psychology and psychiatry*, edited by E. L. Grigorenko. New York: Springer.

Markovic, J. 2012. Criminal justice and public health approaches to violent crime: Complementary perspectives. *Geography and Public Safety* 3(2):1-3.

McDonald, C. C., J. A. Deatrick, N. Kassam-Adams, and T. S. Richmond. 2011. Community violence exposure and positive youth development in urban youth. *Journal of Community Health* 36(6):925-932.

Milam, A. J., S. A. Buggs, C. D. M. Furr-Holden, P. J. Leaf, C. P. Bradshaw, and D. Webster. 2016. Changes in attitudes toward guns and shootings following implementation of the Baltimore Safe Streets Intervention. *Journal of Urban Health* 93(4):609-626.

NASEM (National Academies of Sciences, Engineering, and Medicine). 2015. *Means of violence: Workshop in brief.* Washington, DC: The National Academies Press. https://doi.org/10.17226/21814.

NASEM. 2016a. *Applying a health lens to business practices, policies, and investments: Workshop summary.* Washington, DC: The National Academies Press. https://doi.org/10.17226/21842.

NASEM. 2016b. *Framing the dialogue on race and ethnicity to advance health equity: Proceedings of a workshop.* Washington, DC: The National Academies Press. https://doi.org/0.17226/23576.

Pinderhughes, H., R. A. Davis, and M. Williams. 2015. *Adverse community experiences and resilience: A framework for addressing and preventing community trauma.* Oakland, CA: Prevention Institute.

President's Task Force on 21st Century Policing. 2015. *Final report of the President's Task Force on Policing in the 21st Century.* Washington, DC: Office of Community Oriented Policing Services.

Ransford, C., C. Kane, and G. Slutkin. 2013. Cure violence: A disease control approach to reduce violence and change behavior. In *Epidemiological criminology: Theory to practice,* edited by W. Waltermaurer and T. A. Akers. New York: Routledge. Pp. 232-242.

Sciandra, M., L. Sanbonmatsu, G. J. Duncan, L. A. Gennetian, L. F. Katz, R. C. Kessler, J. R. Kling, and J. Ludwig. 2013. Long-term effects of the moving to opportunity residential mobility experiment on crime and delinquency. *Journal of Experimental Criminology* 9(4):451-489.

South, E. C., M. C. Kondo, R. A. Cheney, and C. C. Branas. 2015. Neighborhood blight, stress, and health: A walking trial of urban greening and ambulatory heart rate. *American Journal of Public Health* 105(5):e1-e5.

Tach, L., S. F. Jacoby, T. Guerra, D. J. Wiebe, and T. S. Richmond. 2016. The effect of microneighborhood conditions on adult educational attainment in a subsidized housing intervention. *Housing Policy Debate* 26(2):380-397. Dx.doi.org/10.1080/10511482.2015.1107118.

Teitelman, A., C. C. McDonald, D. J. Wiebe, N. Thomas, T. Guerra, N. Kassam-Adams, and T. S. Richmond. 2010. Youth's strategies for staying safe and coping with the stress of living in violent communities. *Journal of Community Psychology* 38(7):874-885.

Weinstein, E., J. Wolin, and S. Rose. 2014. *Trauma informed community building: A model for strengthening community in trauma affected neighborhoods.* San Fransico, CA: Health Equity Institute and Bridge Housing. http://bridgehousing.com/PDFs/TICB.Paper5.14.pdf (accessed September 15, 2016).

Williams, T. 2014. Cities mobilize to help those threatened by gentrification. *The New York Times.* http://www.nytimes.com/2014/03/04/us/cities-helping-residents-resist-the-new-gentry.html (accessed November 1, 2016).

Appendix B

Workshop Agenda

Roundtable on Population Health Improvement
Community Violence as a Population Health Issue: A Workshop

June 16, 2016

AGENDA
Location: Lutheran Church of the Good Shepherd
7420 Fourth Avenue, Brooklyn, NY 11209

Workshop Objectives:

1. Explore the impacts of trauma and violence on communities.
2. Explore strategies and approaches that communities and multisector partners are using to prevent violence and build resilience.
3. Explore the evidence base for the effectiveness of these strategies and approaches for reducing the impact of violence on communities.
4. Provide a platform to showcase examples that can serve as models for other communities, with explicit attention to the intersections of structural racism and structural violence.

8:30 am **Welcome and Overview of the Day**

George Isham, senior advisor, HealthPartners; senior fellow, HealthPartners Institute for Education and Research, co-chair, Roundtable on Population Health Improvement

Thomas LaVeist, professor and chair, Milken Institute School of Public Health, The George Washington University; chair, planning committee; member, Roundtable on Population Health Improvement

8:45 am **The Impact of Racism and Violence on Communities**

Speaker: John A. Rich, professor, Drexel University School of Public Health; member, planning committee

9:15 am **Q&A/Discussion**

9:45 am **Break**

10:00 am **Changing Landscapes of Violence Through Social and Physical Interventions**

Moderator: Therese Richmond, Andrea B. Laporte Endowed Professor of Nursing; associate dean for research and innovation, University of Pennsylvania School of Nursing; member, planning committee

Speaker: Howard Pinderhughes, associate professor and chair, social and behavioral sciences, University of California, San Francisco, School of Nursing

Speaker: Charles Branas, professor, biostatistics and epidemiology; director, Penn Injury Science Center; director, Urban Health Lab, Perelman School of Medicine, University of Pennsylvania

10:50 am **Q&A/Discussion**

11:15 am **Local Strategies to Build Community Resilience and Safety**

Moderator: Lourdes Rodríguez, program officer, New York State Health Foundation; member, planning committee; member, Roundtable on Population Health Improvement

Speaker: Roberto Rodríguez, outreach worker supervisor, Stand Up to Violence (SUV), Jacobi Medical Center

Speaker: Devone Boggan, founder and CEO, Advance Peace

12:00 pm **Q&A/Discussion**

12:30 pm **Lunch**

1:30 pm **Evidence of Program and Initiative Impact**

Moderator: Daniel Webster, professor, health policy and management, Johns Hopkins Bloomberg School of Public Health; director, Johns Hopkins Center for Gun Policy and Research; deputy director for research, Johns Hopkins Center for the Prevention of Youth Violence; member, planning committee

Speaker: Jeffrey Butts, director, Research and Evaluation Center, John Jay College of Criminal Justice

Speaker: Thea James, vice president of mission and associate chief medical officer, Boston Medical Center, by WebEx

2:30 pm **Q&A/Discussion**

3:00 pm **Break**

3:15 pm **Public Health–Informed Policing**

Moderator: Ted Corbin, associate professor in the department of emergency medicine, Drexel University School of Medicine; member, planning committee

Speaker: Steve Marans, Harris Professor in the Child Study Center; director, National Center for Children Exposed to Violence/Childhood Violent Trauma Center at the Yale Child Study Center; director, Trauma Service; professor of psychiatry, Yale School of Medicine

Speaker: John Markovic, senior social science analyst, Office of Community Oriented Policing Services (COPS), U.S. Department of Justice

Speaker: Medina Henry, associate director of Training and Technical Assistance, Center for Court Innovation

4:15 pm **Q&A/Discussion**

4:45 pm **Closing Remarks and Reflections on the Day**

Thomas LaVeist, professor and chair, Milken Institute School of Public Health, The George Washington University; chair, planning committee; member, Roundtable on Population Health Improvement

Sanne Magnan, former president and chief executive officer, Institute for Clinical Health Systems; member, workshop planning committee; co-chair, Roundtable on Population Health Improvement

5:15 pm **Adjourn Session**

Appendix C

Biographical Sketches of Workshop Speakers and Moderators

DeVone Boggan serves as founder and CEO of Advance Peace, which disrupts gun violence in U.S. urban neighborhoods. It is a comprehensive, community-driven, developmental strategy that partners with and is informed by those who have the greatest influence on altering the urban gun violence epidemic. Advance Peace provides a unique transformational experience to young men involved in lethal firearm offenses by placing them in a high-touch, personalized Fellowship or what Mr. Boggan has coined as a "blow their minds on *LIFE* Opportunity." Mr. Boggan is the former neighborhood safety director and founding director of the Office of Neighborhood Safety (ONS) for the City of Richmond, California. ONS is a government non–law enforcement agency that is charged with reducing firearm assaults and associated deaths in Richmond. Under his leadership as neighborhood safety director, the city experienced a 75 percent reduction in gun violence between 2007, when ONC was created, and 2015.

Charles C. Branas, Ph.D., is a professor of epidemiology, director of the Penn Injury Science Center, and director of the Urban Health Lab at the University of Pennsylvania. Dr. Branas works to improve health and health care and is recognized for his efforts to reduce violence and enhance emergency care. Much of his work incorporates human geography and place-based interventions. His studies have been replicated nationally and in cities across the United States and other countries. Dr. Branas has served on boards and offered scientific expertise for numerous U.S. groups, including the National Institutes of Health, Centers for Disease

Control and Prevention, and the National Academies of Sciences, Engineering, and Medicine. He has also worked with scientific organizations in Canada, Greece, Guatemala, the Netherlands, New Zealand, and South Africa. The U.S. Supreme Court and the U.S. Congress have cited his work. He is a past president of the Society for Advancement of Violence and Injury Research and an elected member of the American Epidemiological Society. He is currently focused on a series of natural experiments and large randomized controlled field trials that alter urban environments to determine the effects on health and safety in multiple cities.

Jeffrey Butts, Ph.D., is director of the Research and Evaluation Center at John Jay College of Criminal Justice, an adjunct member of the doctoral faculty in the Graduate Center of the City University of New York, and a member of the Science Advisory Board for the Office of Justice Programs in the U.S. Department of Justice. Previously he was a research fellow with Chapin Hall at the University of Chicago and director of the Program on Youth Justice at the Urban Institute. His work focuses on discovering and improving policies and programs for youth involved in the justice system. Since 1990, Dr. Butts has managed more than $18 million of research projects and worked with policy makers and justice practitioners in 28 states and several other countries. He has published two books, dozens of monographs and reports for government agencies and foundations, as well as articles in academic and peer-reviewed journals. His research findings and policy views have been covered by *The New York Times*, *The Washington Post*, *The Los Angeles Times*, *The Economist*, National Public Radio, CBS News, and many other media sources. He began his justice career as a drug and alcohol counselor with the juvenile court in Eugene, Oregon. Dr. Butts is a graduate of the University of Oregon and earned his Ph.D. from the University of Michigan.

Ted Corbin, M.D., M.P.P., is an associate professor in the Department of Emergency Medicine at the Drexel University College of Medicine. He also serves as the founding medical director of "Healing Hurt People," an emergency department–based, trauma-informed intervention strategy for victims of intentional injury at Hahnemann Hospital as well as St. Christopher's Hospital for Children. Dr. Corbin also co-directs the Center for Nonviolence and Social Justice at Drexel University School of Public Health, where he holds a joint appointment. He was awarded a Stoneleigh Foundation Fellowship and an Annie E. Casey Foundation grant to explore the impact of posttraumatic stress disorder on violently injured youth and young adults, and to evaluate the effectiveness of Healing Hurt People. His work focuses broadly on addressing the trauma in the lives of victims of violence, especially boys and men of color for whom violence is a leading cause of disability and death. Dr. Corbin received his B.S. in biology from Lincoln University and his M.D. from Drexel University College of Medicine. He earned his Master of Public Policy from the Woodrow Wilson School at Princeton University. In 2005, he was awarded a Soros Physician Advocacy Fellowship. Dr. Corbin is board certified in emergency medicine. Dr. Corbin provided expert testimony to the Defending Childhood Task Force, charged by Eric Holder, U.S. Attorney General, on his work in violence intervention. Dr. Corbin has also provided practice-based evidence to the National Academy of Medicine on public health approaches to violence intervention.

Rachel Davis, M.S.W., is managing director of the Prevention Institute, playing a key role in advancing the conceptual work of the organization. For the past 10 years with the Prevention Institute, Ms. Davis has developed and overseen projects pertaining to preventing violence, community health and reducing inequity, health care reform, and mental health. She develops tools and materials to support local and state initiatives and trains government agencies, foundations, and community collaboratives across the United States. Ms. Davis also oversees qualitative research and literature reviews and writes extensively. She speaks and consults nationwide on topics related to her fields. Ms. Davis serves as project director for UNITY (Urban Networks to Increase Thriving Youth through Violence Prevention), the Institute's national initiative funded by the Centers for Disease Control and Prevention to strengthen and support the largest U.S. cities in more effectively preventing violence. She also provided research, script development, facilitator training, and management expertise to the Institute's Partnerships for Preventing Violence satellite series, which trained more than 15,000 leaders and practitioners across the country. Ms. Davis has facilitated planning processes for various city and county governments, helping them to generate strategic action frameworks for preventing violence. She is the advisory board chair for the California Cities Gang Prevention Network.

Amanda Geller, Ph.D., M.Eng., is a clinical associate professor of sociology and the director of the M.A. program in Applied Quantitative Research at New York University. Dr. Geller's research examines the interactions between criminal justice policy and socioeconomic disadvantage and their joint effects on urban neighborhoods, families, and individuals. She focuses specifically on the role of parental incarceration in families, and the administration of justice related to police–public interactions. Her work has been published in outlets that reach the diverse constituencies with interest in the criminal justice system, including the *Journal of Empirical Legal Studies*, *Demography*, the *Journal of Marriage and Family*, and the

American Journal of Public Health. In the summer of 2013, she presented at a White House workshop on parental incarceration convened by the American Bar Foundation.

Medina Henry, M.P.A., is associate director of training and technical assistance at the Center for Court Innovation. In this role, she provides consulting services to jurisdictions around the nation, including assistance provided under the Problem-Solving Justice Initiative of the Bureau of Justice Assistance at the U.S. Department of Justice (DOJ). The Problem-Solving Justice Initiative seeks to promote the use of problem-solving practices in an effort to reduce crime and incarceration while strengthening public trust in justice. Ms. Henry also spearheads technical assistance for nine sites funded by the Minority Youth Violence Prevention initiative, a collaboration between the Office of Minority Health at the U.S. Department of Health and Human Services and the Office of Community Oriented Policing Services at DOJ. She began her career at the Center shortly after earning her M.P.A. at Baruch College. Ms. Henry started as the program coordinator for the Center's AmeriCorps program and was promoted to planner for the Red Hook Community Justice Center. While in Red Hook, she helped the Justice Center to plan and launch the Red Hook Responders, a social service program focused on addressing the community's needs after Hurricane Sandy; Red Hook CARES, which provides crisis support and case management to survivors of violence; and a host of other projects.

George Isham, M.D., M.S., is senior advisor to HealthPartners, responsible for working with the board of directors and the senior management team on health and quality of care improvement for patients, members, and the community. Dr. Isham is also Senior Fellow, HealthPartners Research Foundation and facilitates forward progress at the intersection of population health research and public policy. Dr. Isham is active nationally and currently co-chairs the National Quality Forum–convened Measurement Application Partnership, chairs the National Committee for Quality Assurance's (NCQA's) clinical program committee, and is a member of NCQA's committee on performance measurement. He is a former member of the Centers for Disease Control and Prevention's (CDC's) Task Force on Community Preventive Services and the Agency for Healthcare Research and Quality's U.S. Preventive Services Task Force. He currently serves on the advisory committee to the director of CDC. His practice experience as a general internist was with the U.S. Navy, at the Freeport Clinic in Freeport, Illinois, and as a clinical assistant professor of medicine at the University of Wisconsin Hospitals and Clinics in Madison, Wisconsin. In 2014 Dr. Isham was elected to the National

Academy of Medicine. He is a past chair of the Health and Medicine Division's (HMD's) Roundtable on Health Literacy and has chaired three studies in addition to serving on a number of HMD studies related to health and quality of care. In 2003 Dr. Isham was appointed as a lifetime National Associate of the National Academy of Sciences in recognition of his contributions to the work of the HMD.

Thea James, M.D., is an associate professor of emergency medicine at Boston University School of Medicine. She is vice president of mission and associate chief medical officer at Boston Medical Center and a past president of the medical and dental staff at Boston Medical Center. She is an assistant dean in the Office of Diversity and Multicultural Affairs, and the director of the Violence Intervention Advocacy Program at Boston Medical Center. Dr. James is a founding member of the National Network of Hospital-Based Violence Intervention Advocacy Programs (NNHVIP). She serves on the Steering Committee and the Research Working Group of NNHVIP. In 2011, Dr. James was appointed to Attorney General Eric Holder's National Task Force on Children Exposed to Violence. The task force report was released and presented to the Attorney General in 2012. Dr. James is member of the Boards of Blue Cross Blue Shield Foundation and the Heller School at Brandeis University. She has chaired and served on national committees within the Society for Academic Emergency Medicine (SAEM). She was appointed to the SAEM Women in Academic Emergency Medicine Task Force. Dr. James served on the Massachusetts Board of Registration in Medicine from 2009 to 2012, when she served as chair of the Licensing Committee. Dr. James is the 2008 awardee of the Boston Public Health Commission's Mulligan Award for public service. In 2012, she was a recipient of the Suffolk County District Attorney's Role Model Award. In 2012, the Boston Business Journal honored Dr. James with its Health Care Hero Award. She was the 2014 recipient of the Schwartz Center Compassionate Care Award. In 2015, the Boston Chamber of Commerce awarded Dr. James with the Pinnacle Award, which honors women in business and the professions. She was selected by Atlanta Victim Assistance Inc. to receive the 2016 Barney L. Simms "Trailblazer" Award in June 2016. Dr. James is a supervising medical officer on the Boston Disaster Medical Assistance Team, which has responded to several U.S. and global disasters, including 9/11 and Hurricane Katrina. In 2006, Dr. James and a colleague co-founded Unified for Global Healing. The organization takes multidisciplinary teams to Africa, India, and Haiti, where they work with local partners to conduct sustainable projects. She is a member of the Board of Directors of Equal Health, formerly called Physicians for Haiti. A graduate of Georgetown University School of Medicine, Dr. James trained in emergency medicine at Boston City Hospital, where she was a chief resident. Board Certified in emergency medicine, she has been the recipient of the Outstanding Faculty Award at Boston University School of Medicine's Department of Emergency Medicine, and has twice received the Department of Emergency Medicine Chair's Award.

Thomas A. LaVeist, Ph.D., is chair of the Department of Health Policy and Management at The George Washington University (GW) Milken Institute School of Public Health. He joined GW after 25 years on the faculty of the Johns Hopkins Bloomberg School of Public Health, where he was the William C. and Nancy F. Richardson Professor in Health Policy and director of the Hopkins Center for Health Disparities Solutions. He received his Bachelor's Degree from the University of Maryland Eastern Shore and his Doctorate in Medical Sociology from the University of Michigan. He completed his Postdoctoral Fellowship in Public Health at the Michigan School of Public Health. Dr. LaVeist has published more than 100 articles in scientific journals. In addition to his scholarly writing, Dr. LaVeist has written articles for *Newsweek* Magazine, *Black Enterprise* Magazine, and *The Baltimore Sun*. He is a highly sought after lecturer at leading universities, corporations, professional conferences, and workshops. His research has been funded by the National Institutes of Health (NIH), Centers for Disease Control and Prevention, U.S. Department of Defense, Commonwealth Fund, Sage Foundation, and Agency for Healthcare Research and Quality. In 2012 he organized and hosted the International Conference on Health in the African Diaspora, which brought together health advocates from 24 countries in the Western Hemisphere. Dr. LaVeist has provided consultation services for numerous federal agencies and health care organizations on minority health and cultural competency issues and racial disparities in health. His dissertation on racial disparities in infant mortality was awarded the 1989 Roberta G. Simmons Outstanding Dissertation Award by the American Sociological Association. He is the recipient of the "Innovation Award" from NIH, and the "Knowledge Award" from the U.S. Department of Health and Human Services Office of Minority Health. In 2013 he was elected to membership in the National Academy of Medicine. The second edition of his edited volume *Race, Ethnicity and Health: A Public Health Reader* (Jossey-Bass Publishers) was published in 2012. His textbook *Minority Populations and Health: An Introduction to Race, Ethnicity and Health in the United States* (Jossey-Bass) was published in 2005. He is also the author of *The DayStar Guide to Colleges for African American Students* (Stanley Kaplan/Simon and Schuster), and co-author of *8 Steps to Help Black Families Pay for College* (Princeton Review/Random House). His most recent book project, *Legacy of the Crossing: Slavery, Race, and Contemporary Health in the African Diaspora*, is planned for publication in 2017.

Sanne Magnan, M.D., Ph.D., is the co-chair of the Roundtable on Population Health Improvement. Dr. Magnan served as president and CEO of the Institute for Clinical Systems Improvement (ICSI) until January 2016. From 2007 until 2010, she was commissioner of health for the Minnesota Department of Health, an appointment by former Minnesota Governor Tim Pawlenty. She had significant responsibility for implementation of Minnesota's 2008 health reform legislation, including the Statewide Health Improvement Program, standardized quality reporting, development of provider peer grouping, certification process for health care homes, and baskets of care. She returned as ICSI's president and CEO in 2011. Dr. Magnan also currently serves as a staff physician at the Tuberculosis Clinic at St. Paul-Ramsey County Department of Public Health and as a clinical assistant professor of medicine at the University of Minnesota. Her experience also includes serving as vice president and medical director of Consumer Health at Blue Cross and Blue Shield of Minnesota, where she was responsible for case management, disease management, and consumer engagement. Dr. Magnan holds an M.D. and a Ph.D. in medicinal chemistry from the University of Minnesota, and is a board certified internist. She earned her bachelor's degree in pharmacy from the University of North Carolina. She has served on the Board of Minnesota Community Measurement, and the Board of NorthPoint Health & Wellness Center, a federally qualified health center and part of Hennepin Health. She was named 1 of the 100 Influential Health Care Leaders by *Minnesota Physician* magazine in 2004, 2008, and 2012. Since 2012, she has participated in the Process Redesign Advisory Group for the National Center for Interprofessional Practice and Education coordinated through the University of Minnesota. Recently, she became a Senior Fellow, HealthPartners Institute for Education and Research. She is participating in several Technical Expert Panels for the Centers for Medicare & Medicaid Services on population health measures, and is a member of the Population-based Payment Workgroup of the Healthcare Payment Learning and Action Network. She is also on the Interdisciplinary Application/Translation Committee of the Interdisciplinary Association for Population Health Sciences.

Steven Marans, Ph.D., M.S.W., is the Harris Professor of Child Psychoanalysis and professor of Psychiatry at the Child Study Center and Department of Psychiatry, Yale University School of Medicine, and is a child and adult psychoanalyst. Dr. Marans is the director of the Childhood Violent Trauma Center and the founder of the Child Development-Community Policing (CD-CP) Program. Begun in 1991, it is a national model for collaborative responses of mental health and law enforcement professionals to children and families exposed to violence that occurs in homes, neighborhoods, and schools. Dr. Marans is also the co-developer of the Child and Family Traumatic Stress Intervention, an evidence-based, brief early intervention that decreases the development of longer term posttraumatic disorders in children who have been impacted by recent trauma. Among his writings, Dr. Marans co-authored *The Police–Mental Health Partnership: A Community-Based Response to Urban Violence* based on the CD-CP experience and, in 2005, a book titled *Listening to Fear: Helping Kids Cope, from Nightmares to the Nightly News*. Dr. Marans served on the U.S. Attorney General's National Task Force on Children Exposed to Violence and is a co-author of the task force's report.

John Markovic, M.A., is a senior social science analyst in the Research and Development Division at the U.S. Department of Justice (DOJ) Office of Community Oriented Policing Services (COPS). His responsibilities include grant management and maintaining a substantive focus on multiple issue areas, including urban violence, gangs, the use of geographic information systems (GIS) to promote public safety, homeland security, and police communications and technology. He has actively participated in DOJ-wide initiatives and other federal partnerships, including the Violence Reduction Network, the Gang Research Evidence Integration Team, a Geospatial Technology Working Group, and an innovative grant collaboration supported by COPS and the U.S. Department of Health and Human Services Office of Minority Health. Prior to joining COPS, Markovic was a program manager at the International Association of Chiefs of Police, managing work on broad-ranging topic areas, including crime mapping and geospatial analysis; juvenile justice; civil rights; and promoting diversity in policing. Mr. Markovic's other experience includes applied research and geographic information system analysis at the Vera Institute of Justice in New York, the Project on Human Development in Chicago Neighborhoods, and Mount Sinai Hospital of Chicago, where he conducted research in a unique Pediatric Ecology Program engaged in medical/legal assessments of alleged cases of child abuse and neglect. Mr. Markovic's current research focuses on public health approaches to violence reduction, as well as the use of social network analysis to promote targeted intervention to reduce violence. Mr. Markovic holds an M.A. in criminal justice from the University of Illinois at Chicago.

Howard Pinderhughes, Ph.D., is an associate professor in the Department of Social and Behavioral Sciences, University of California, San Francisco, School of Nursing. Dr. Pinderhughes is the author of *Race in the Hood: Conflict and Violence Among Urban Youth*, which examined the dynamics of racial violence in New York City. His forthcoming book, *Dealing With Danger: How Inner City Youth Cope with the Violence That Surrounds Them,* examines the production of youth violence and how urban adolescents think about, experience, and make decisions about the use of violence. Additionally, he served as the co-principal investigator for the Center on Culture, Immigration and Youth Violence Prevention, one of the Centers for Disease Control and Prevention's Academic Centers of Excellence in Youth Violence Prevention.

John A. Rich, M.D., M.P.H., is a professor at the Drexel University School of Public Health. He has been a leader in the field of public health, and his work has focused on serving one of the nation's most ignored and underserved populations—African American men in urban settings. In 2006, Dr. Rich was granted a MacArthur Foundation Fellowship. In awarding this distinction, the Foundation cited his work to design "new models of health care that stretch across the boundaries of public health, education, social service, and justice systems to engage young men in caring for themselves and their peers." Prior to Drexel University, Dr. Rich served as the medical director of the Boston Public Health Commission. As a primary care doctor at Boston Medical Center, Dr. Rich created the Young Men's Health Clinic and initiated the Boston HealthCREW, a program to train inner city young men to become peer health educators who focus on the health of men and boys in their communities. He earned his Dartmouth A.B. in English, his M.D. from Duke University Medical School, and his master's from the Harvard School of Public Health. He completed his internship and residency at the Massachusetts General Hospital and was a fellow in general internal medicine at Harvard Medical School. He received an honorary Doctor of Science degree from Dartmouth in 2007 and now serves on its Board of Trustees. In 2009, Dr. Rich was inducted into the National Academy of Medicine. His recently published book about urban violence, *Wrong Place, Wrong Time: Trauma and Violence in the Lives of Young Black Men*, has drawn critical acclaim.

Therese S. Richmond, Ph.D., FAAN, CRNP, is the Andrea B. Laporte Professor of Nursing and associate dean for research and innovation at the University of Pennsylvania (Penn) School of Nursing. Dr. Richmond's research interests focus on injury and violence. She has an extensive body of research aimed to improve outcomes after injury and she addresses the interaction between physical injury and the postinjury psychological consequences. This work has helped to identify groups of injured patients most likely to experience suboptimal outcomes and points to screening and interventions to improve those outcomes. Dr. Richmond has been funded by the National Institute of Mental Health to examine the effects of developing depression and posttraumatic stress disorder (PTSD) following injury on disability and quality of life, and she developed a predictive screener to identify those patients at highest risk for the future emergence of postinjury depression and PTSD. She is currently funded by the National Institute of Nursing Research to examine psychological consequences of serious injury in urban African American men. Dr. Richmond conducts studies to prevent violence and to reduce its impact on individuals, families, and communities. She co-founded the Firearm & Injury Center at Penn and directs the Training, Education & Outreach Core of the Penn Injury Science Center. She is committed to community-based participatory research and interdisciplinary partnerships. She co-directs a National Institutes of Health-Fogarty Training Grant to train injury and violence scientists in Guatemala. Dr. Richmond's research contributions have been recognized by the American Association of Critical Care Nurses (AACN) Excellence in Research Award, and the AACN General Electric Healthcare Pioneering Spirit Award for her research in firearm injuries and violence. She has been inducted into the Sigma Theta Tau International Nurse Researcher Hall of Fame.

Lourdes Rodríguez, Dr.P.H., M.P.H., is a program officer for the New York State Health Foundation (NYSHealth) on projects related to building healthy communities. In this capacity, she works toward supporting neighborhood-level interventions to increase healthy food options and improve the built environment; advancing public policies that promote healthy living; and increasing access to programs that help New Yorkers lead healthier lives. She also works to support the Foundation's goals to advance primary care, especially on projects aimed to address social determinants of health. Prior to joining NYSHealth, Dr. Rodríguez served as the associate director of community partnerships for the Healthy Neighborhoods initiative at City Harvest. In this position, she oversaw the implementation of the organization's community engagement activities to help address the epidemics of diabetes, cardiovascular disease, and other diet-related diseases in five low-income neighborhoods of New York City. From 2004 to 2012, she was on the faculty of the Columbia University Mailman School of Public Health. She currently holds an appointment as adjunct associate professor at the New York University Global Institute of Public Health. In 2011, she co-edited a book examining community mobilization for health, and has authored numerous publications on the subjects of violence prevention, health of vulnerable populations, mental health, community mobilization, and active living. Dr. Rodríguez received a B.S. in industrial biotechnology from the Mayagüez Campus of the University of Puerto Rico, an M.P.H. from the University of Connecticut, and a Dr.P.H. from Columbia University's Mailman School of Public Health. She serves on the board of Inwood Community Services, Inc., and on the consensus group of City Life Is Moving Bodies (CLIMB), a neighborhood-based initiative that plans Hike the Heights, an annual northern Manhattan community mobilization event.

Roberto Rodríguez is a native of the Bronx. At the age of 17, his poor decisions and participation in high-risk activity led to a 16-year prison sentence. While incarcerated, Mr. Rodríguez went through a deep transformation, which developed his positive outlook on life. He is now employed at the Jacobi Medical Center's Stand Up to Violence (SUV) program as an outreach supervisor. In this role, he strives to prevent young men and women from engaging in high-risk activity and repeating the mistakes he made. His experience gives him credibility with young adults and makes him a powerful messenger. As a supervisor, Mr. Rodríguez's continued success after being released from prison more than 7 years ago is an inspiration for the program's employees, most of whom are currently navigating the difficult reentry process. Mr. Rodríguez was previously employed at Fortune Society, a nonprofit organization that works with the formerly incarcerated. He has also achieved great success and notoriety training dogs as companions for disabled veterans with posttraumatic stress disorder. In 2011, he was featured on OWN (the Oprah Winfrey Network) for his participation in the Puppies Behind Bars program. Mr. Rodríguez is currently pursuing a bachelor's degree in liberal arts at The College of New Rochelle.

Daniel W. Webster, Sc.D., M.P.H., is a professor of health policy and management at the Johns Hopkins Bloomberg School of Public Health. Dr. Webster is director of the Johns Hopkins Center for Gun Policy and Research, deputy director for research for the Johns Hopkins Center for the Prevention of Youth Violence, and core faculty of the Johns Hopkins Center for Injury Research and Policy. Dr. Webster holds a joint appointment as professor in the School of Education's Division of Public Safety Leadership at Johns Hopkins. Dr. Webster is one of the nation's leading experts on firearm policy and the prevention of gun violence. He is co-editor of *Reducing Gun Violence in America: Informing Policy with Evidence and Analysis* (JHU Press, 2013). He has published numerous articles on firearm policy, youth gun acquisition and carrying, the prevention of gun violence, intimate partner violence, and adolescent violence prevention. He has studied the effects of a variety of violence prevention interventions, including state firearm and alcohol policies, policing strategies, street outreach and conflict mediation, public education campaigns, and school-based curricula. Dr. Webster teaches Understanding and Preventing Violence; Research and Evaluation Methods for Health Policy; and a Graduate Seminar in Health and Public Policy.